WORK's a WE THING™

DANNY McCALL

TalentSphere Academy Press
USA

Publisher's Cataloging-in-Publication Data
McCall, Danny.
Work's a We Thing / Danny McCall.
p. cm.
ISBN 978-0-9718122-1-5
1. Job satisfaction—Fiction. 2. Occupations—Fiction. 3. Organizational effectiveness—Fiction.
PS3613.C34514 W67 2008
813—dc22   2008908960

TalentSphere, LLC
The Atrium
1225 Weisgarber Road, Suite 370
Knoxville, Tennessee 37909
Tel: (865) 546-4990
inquiries@talentsphere.com
WWT-v5-052212

A relationship, I think, is like a shark, you know? It has to constantly move forward or it dies. And I think what we got on our hands is a dead shark.
— Woody Allen

A bizarre sensation pervades a relationship of pretense. No truth seems true. A simple morning's greeting and response appear loaded with innuendo and fraught with implications. Each nicety becomes more sterile and each withdrawal more permanent.
— Maya Angelou

The greatest secrets are written on billboards.
— Daniel Quinn

CONTENTS

"Inspiration is not the exclusive privilege of poets or artists. There is, there has been, there will always be a certain group of people whom inspiration visits. It's made up of all those who've consciously chosen their calling and do their job with love and imagination. It may include doctors, teachers, gardeners—I could list a hundred more professions. Their work becomes one continuous adventure as long as they manage to keep discovering new challenges in it. Difficulties and setbacks never quell their curiosity. A swarm of new questions emerges from every problem that they solve. Whatever inspiration is, it's born from a continuous "I don't know."

There aren't many such people. Most of the earth's inhabitants work to get by. They work because they have to. They didn't pick this or that kind of job out of passion; the circumstances of their lives did the choosing for them. Loveless work, boring work, work valued only because others haven't got even that much—this is one of the harshest human miseries. And there's no sign that coming centuries will produce any changes for the better as far as this goes."

— Wislawa Szymborska
Nobel Lecture, December 7, 1996
Stockholm

ONE

CALAMITY

A brilliant, crisp spring morning illuminated her kitchen windows. Cynthia slowly drank the first cup of coffee of the day. Another Monday filled with the same old dread she had felt for months. It was her job.

Dale, her husband, moving perfectly on the tracks of his daily routine, was heading out the door after feeding the dog. He looked at her. He saw the same troublesome expression he had come to know so well that had shaped her face lately. He stopped and offered with a cautious, well-intended tone, "You don't have to stay there, you know. There are plenty of other places that would be eager to have your skills and experience."

"Yeh, I know, but I really don't know what I want to do or where I want to do it," Cynthia responded. "I only know that my work makes me miserable and it's beginning to spread like a big ugly cloud into all the corners of my life.

 I really don't know what's wrong. I feel paralyzed, like I don't even know myself or my true desires anymore. I used to be so eager to go to work each day. I miss that. It was a really good feeling. My work is important to me. I like who I work with, but it's just not making me happy lately. I just don't know why I feel so lost."

Dale's concern had grown over the last few weeks. Cynthia's funk and dark moods related to work seemed more serious. They were beginning to impact their relationship in many ways. He felt helpless. He too had problems at work from time to time, but he just accepted this as the way it was. Anyhow, he certainly did not have any background in career counseling or psychology.

As Dale left the room, back on the rails of his morning routine, he gave her a kiss and said, "You've had these bad feelings for a long time. You're looking at the classifieds every Sunday and spending a lot of time on the job boards in the evenings. It's not getting any better, so you might want to begin taking action. I realize you're scared to share your true feelings with your boss. I would be too, for that just complicates things. Maybe you should at least send out a few resumes for the jobs that seem interesting, have a few interviews and see what happens."

Now passing through the kitchen door, he looked back, "Hey, what about talking with Elli about your issues this afternoon? She's so passionate about her work lately that it seems almost weird."

"Maybe. I don't want to bother her with my problems, or as you say, my 'issues.'"

"Sorry, I did not mean anything with that word. It was just an idea. I'm not trying to be pushy. Anyway, do whatever it takes. I'm behind you in whatever you want to do! I'm sorry I can't help more. Love ya!" And Dale was out the door.

Prosperity is a great teacher; adversity a greater.
— William Hazzlitt

Eleanor (Elli) and Cynthia had been best friends since high school. They had always freely shared their life joys and tribulations with each other, including supporting each other through more than a few tough, sometimes "interesting" situations. Though both had been married for quite a while, they continued to keep their close bonds. They made it a point to meet every couple of weeks after work to chat. They had such a meeting planned for today at a local coffee shop next to Cynthia's gym. What Dale had said was true. Elli loved her work. She had advanced rapidly in her organization and in the last year or so, appeared to be one of the rising stars there. Cynthia assumed that Elli's success and joy from her work had been simply the right combination of skills, place, timing … and perhaps most importantly, luck.

On her commute this morning, Cynthia reflected on the "good old days" at work before the confusion, constant changes, increased workload and all the new people coming and going. It seemed as if nothing she did lately was the right thing, or was done fast enough, if it got done at all, to suit the demands coming at her from every direction. In fact, with all the shifting priorities taking place, she was often unsure what she was actually supposed to be doing. She always seemed to be focused on just the opposite of what her supervisor, Rick, desired from her. However, she generally learned of this only after the fact by his subtle, indirect or cryptic comments.

She was trying earnestly to perform well, but despite her best intentions, what she was doing was turning out wrong too often. Her attention was scattered in too many directions and the chaos only seemed to grow greater with each passing day. Strangely enough, even in the midst of what seemed to be constant craziness in her job recently, she actually felt a little bored, restless and detached. She used to feel more a part of her work. Yet in spite of all this, for some reason, she did not want to leave her organization. There was something special about the place and what they did that she liked. When work was good, it gave her a sense of purpose and meaning in her life that was important to her. How could she possibly make any sense of all of this? It seemed too complicated.

In the middle of difficulty lies opportunity.
— Albert Einstein

As usual, Cynthia quickly climbed the four flights of stairs to her department, avoiding the elevator. She walked down the hall to her area, tossed her sweater on the back of a chair and made a dash for her department's coffee pot.

She found Gerald stirring his coffee. He turned and looked at her. For an instant, she saw an expression on Gerald's face that alerted her that something was troubling him. She and Gerald had both been hired the same month many years ago. They had been on many of the same teams and projects. Though now in different work groups, they remained close friends at work. They had met many impossible deadlines together and had performed their share of miracles together in moments of desperation. They were battle-tested. Gerald's face and mind always worked together just like a goldfish bowl—the outside always perfectly revealed the inside.

"What's up?" she quizzed.

"Good morning, Cynthia. You look nice and spring-like today in that bright yellow dress!" he responded with no small amount of energy.

"Thanks Gerald. Good deflect, but what's the reason for the look on that face of yours?"

"What look?"

"The one you're now hiding so well."

"Nothing, just a long weekend," Gerald responded, again trying to bounce the topic in another direction and then get away as quickly as possible.

"Come on buddy. We've been miners in this salt mine too long for secrets," as she humorously nudged with an elbow, then exercised a mock shoveling action.

Gerald didn't know what to do, so he just blurted out what he knew. "The buzz is that you're going to be terminated."

At first Cynthia thought it was a cruel Monday morning joke, but she knew that Gerald never joked, at least not like this. She felt a cold shock wave quickly move through her.

"What? ... When? ... Why?" ... She slowly, forcefully responded, each single-word question tossed at Gerald with the energy of a lobbed cannonball.

 "I have no idea except there have been other rumors that you've been distracted and no longer have the enthusiasm for your work." He paused and then added, "Having worked with you before, I discounted that there was any truth to that."

"What?" Cynthia exclaimed, "I'm just as committed to my work as anyone else here!"

"I know you are, but that's all I know. Honest! There are a couple of people in my group who somehow overheard Rick sharing something about this Friday on the phone with someone. I don't know any details, but considering the sources, I think it's credible." Gerald said this while lowering his voice and avoiding eye contact with her. Clearly he was very uncomfortable. As he turned to walk out, he looked back, "I'm sorry Cynthia, but it seems like you should have at least a little heads up on this. Maybe I should have just kept my mouth shut. Please don't share this with anyone. Neither you nor I are supposed to know this. After all, none of this may be true. This all may be grapevine fertilizer."

Cynthia had no response and let him walk away. Her legs were weak and her heart was pounding. Sure, only moments ago, she was frustrated with her job, but she had at least felt secure. She thought the decision about going or staying was only hers to make, when and if she decided to do so. Now the world had turned upside down and was suddenly spinning out of control. She instantly launched into high anxiety about the prospects of losing her job. What should she do now? She went back to her work area, everything in a bit of slow motion, as they always seem to be during the really bad events in one's life. In fact, she remembered feeling like this right before an automobile accident when she was a teenager. Now, like then, there seemed no avoiding the inevitable, no matter how hard she pressed on the brakes or turned the steering wheel, the car just kept skidding toward the awaiting guardrail.

She had to talk with Rick, her department's supervisor, now! But how would she do this without ratting on Gerald? Maybe she would just do a little verbal song and dance with Rick to see if she could pick up at least some clues. Clues? Heck, he might fire her on the spot! Fearing the worst, Cynthia called his assistant.

"Sorry Cynthia, Rick's out at an off-site all day. Is there anything I can help you with, or would you like to leave a message on his voice mail?" his assistant responded in a very friendly and helpful, but detached manner.

"No, that's fine, I'll just talk with him tomorrow," Cynthia responded.

With a slight tremor in her hands, she next dialed Dale's cell phone. She had to speak with someone. Afterward, she would get to her work. It was going to be a long day. It was good that she had time already planned with Elli later. She really needed to talk.

Home is where one starts from. As we grow older the world becomes stranger, the pattern more complicated.
— T.S. Eliot

TWO

SYNCING

C ynthia arrived at the coffee shop a little early, eager to dump a long day of fretting and lots of worries onto her best friend. She was ready for a caring ear and a sympathetic heart. However, she knew from plenty of past experiences that Elli would not let her wallow in misery nor play host to her pity party. Elli was a "tough love" buddy. She was a real life action hero figure who had no tolerance for whiners.

Most of the time, Cynthia thought that she had a similar personality, at least the one she projected to others. But she then admitted to herself—maybe not so much when she was the one with the problem.

Elli drove up with her new convertible's top down and parked right outside the window where Cynthia was already seated and waiting. Elli immediately saw Cynthia sitting at the window-side table and waved. The sun's bright reflection on the plate glass hid a telling expression on Cynthia's face from Elli. Quickly walking into the coffee shop, Elli broadcasted one of her trademark ear-to-ear smiles.

"Hey girl, can you believe this fine weather? How ya doing? Am I late?" Elli greeted, the smile still radiating upbeat vibes.

Long ago, Cynthia mastered keeping up with Elli's machine gun questions. She instantly compiled her answers, "It's really nice, especially after the winter we've had. OK, I've had better. Nope, I was early."

"What's wrong, buddy? No lottery win today? No roses for no reason from Dale? No dragon-slaying victories at work? Monday blues? None of the above?" Elli was in her normal fine form.

"I'm gonna be fired," Cynthia blurted out in an exaggerated moan, trying to toss a bucket of cold water upon Elli's perky enthusiasm.

"Yeh, right! And I'm now a candidate for president! Wanna be my veep? I think we could have some serious good times in the White House. Whoa, and what about Air Force One parties?"

"Well, I guess I might be available."

"You're serious?" Elli replied, half statement, half question. Her brilliant smile was fast disappearing as she rapidly morphed into "caring friend mode."

"… U h … h u h," Cynthia drew out again, slowly and perfectly for maximum drama coupled with a well-constructed facial pout for the full effect.

"That's impossible. How could anyone with intelligence above a reptile not be begging you to stay with them?"

"I guess you'd need to talk to Rick about that."

"Why? When did you find out? How did they tell you? Does Dale know? What are you going to do?"

"Well, I'm not actually sure it's true, but a friend at work told me today that he had good sources and reasons to believe it's going to happen. Yep, called Dale today. He loves me and he cares, but he's clueless on this stuff. For that matter, so am I."

"So we're only talking rumor mill fodder. Let me guess, you're now in full panic and overreacting without any real evidence?"

"Maybe. Maybe not. 1 know I was really unhappy about work long before I even learned about this. I've been discouraged about my job for months. This is just a new big ol' log that's breaking this camel's back," Cynthia shared, obviously not at all sure what the truth of the matter was.

"Let's sort this out."

"Let's!" Cynthia replied with ample sarcasm.

"Are you and Rick in agreement?"

"Agreement? About what? What are you talking about?"

Elli responded apologetically, "I'm sorry, I keep forgetting you guys don't practice *Relationship Performance™ or RP™* as we call it. I just take it for granted that nowadays everyone's using *RP*."

"You mean that stuff you guys are doing at work that you were raving endlessly about at last year's Christmas party with the girls? Talk about wrong place, wrong topic!"

"Yep, I suppose I was a little too exuberant for the setting. But I still am, maybe even more so. It's nifty. RP has been like a slingshot for me at work, putting me where I want to be."

"Nifty? I haven't heard that since we were giggling together in high school. Sorry, maybe I wasn't paying close attention at the party, for reasons that you may or may not recall, when you were raving before about whatever it is you're raving about now, again. Anyhow, what's so nifty about it?" Cynthia had placed distinct emphasis on "raving" and even more emphasis on "nifty" for impact.

At least she was momentarily distracted by sparring with Elli. That always provided temporary pain relief.

"OK, my skeptical and inattentive friend," Elli said. "Once more, it's called **Relationship Performance ... RP** for short. You use it to understand the forces at play in a workplace. Then you apply it to your advantage with better thought, preparation and dialog to reach shared agreement with your supervisor, or in RP-speak, your *Talent Steward™*.

Yeh, I know it may sound a little corny, cheesy or clichéd at first, but it's the first real, usable and practical approach that really gets to the heart of what every worker and organization needs. It's all upside, no downside. It reveals realities about our work and career that most of us can't typically see without some help."

"So big deal. It also sounds like academic, abstract gobbledy-gook. What's in it for me?" Cynthia jumped in with impatience.

"It keeps you out of trouble at work. Even more importantly, RP improves your insights and gives you a stronger voice to get what you deserve, including being happier at work. RP works at work!"

"Friend, methinks you've been brainwashed. Spare me please! I've got coffee already. I don't need to drink the Kool Aid." Cynthia couldn't help being caustic. Elli's positive energy was affecting her brain like long fingernails slowly playing upon a chalkboard. She had already had enough of this upbeat momentum. After all, she had just 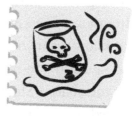 learned she was losing her job. This was no day for motivational speeches. It was probably too late, anyway. Cynthia was determined to be the center of attention, at least this afternoon, with Elli. It was time for a friend's sympathy. This was not a time for learning a new theory, and certainly not a theory about work.

Elli bounced back, not so much defensively or bragging, as just lobbing the facts, "Well, if I'm brainwashed, I'm a programmed zombie who's laughing with fat monthly payroll deposits and a corner office!"

It was true that their careers had taken two very different paths over the last year or so. Elli did not want to bring more attention to the glaring differences between them at work. Especially not now. Elli knew Cynthia was hurting. Maybe she had gone too far.

Cynthia felt like she had been hit in the head with a brick. She tried to hide the blow by looking into her cup, but there was no help to be found there.

Silence.

More silence.

Elli sipped her dark Colombian blend of the day, looking away, out the window into the sunny suburban afternoon. She knew better than to say anything. She did not know what to say, anyway. She was now suspecting she had said way too much or at least spoken with an edge that was too sharp. She hoped that she had not unintentionally crossed over that well-known line.

Cynthia was pensive. After a momentary, deep reality check, she spurted, "Sorry, you didn't deserve that Elli. I'm happy for you. I truly am."

Then she added, "OK, I need help. I admit it. If you know anything that can help me, I'm willing to listen. I'm flailing around in the dark, lost, helpless and without any idea what's going on with my job, or myself for that matter.

I actually don't have a clue what's on Rick's mind about me. I'm not even sure what's taking place in my own mind."

Then, trying to put a little humor back into play, Cynthia pushed back from the table and stood up with a model's straight poise. She looked out the window, hands at her sides and spoke in an uncharacteristic monotone to an invisible 12-step program audience outdoors, "My name is Cynthia. I have a problem. What's more—I may even have an 'issue.'"

Others in the coffee shop took notice of her public admission, though all tried, ineffectively, not to be seen doing so. Cynthia sat back down.

A slight smile, though maybe forced, was emerging on her face.

There are moments when everything is going well,
don't be frightened, it won't last.
— Jules Renard

Idealism increases in direct proportion to one's
distance from the problem.
— John Galsworthy

Getting fired is nature's way of telling you that you
had the wrong job in the first place.
— Hal Lancaster

THREE

PURGING TOXINS

W ith Cynthia's sudden shift in receptiveness, Elli pounced. She hadn't always been able to rise to the occasion in the past, but this time she was confident she could be a big help to her friend.

Elli began, "There's no reason at all to beat yourself up about feeling lost or confused. When it comes to work, we're all lost! When I was first exposed to Relationship Performance, I was surprised how much I misunderstood. Regardless of our education and experience, we're all incredibly illiterate at managing our careers and understanding organizations. For that matter, even understanding what we personally need from our work can be challenging. Prior to RP, we were not taught the way work actually works. Ignorance can be bliss for a short while, but in the long term, ignorance debilitates and creates insecure and dangerous career situations."

Cynthia replied, "I really thought I had a pretty good idea how things work at work. After all, I've got more than a decade of hard-earned experience behind me. I'm sure lost lately. I didn't see my job being in jeopardy at all. I was blind-sided today!"

Elli counseled, "Well, before RP, I was confident I knew all the work ropes. I admit that I also viewed work with a slightly negative slant. I always thought it was sorta the right thing for me to do to rage against the machine. I saw myself as just another David-like worker bee plotting and defending my own interests as best I could against the Goliaths who owned and ran the hive. I saw it as 'me versus them.' Now I know that perspective is wrong and counter-productive."

"Wrong? That way of thinking sounds right-on to me, especially today!" Cynthia argued.

"Well, being helpless wasn't doing anything good for me," Elli confided.

"You? Helpless?" Cynthia doubted that Elli was ever helpless.

"Yep, me," Elli confessed. "You'd be surprised how much I can recall feelings like you may be having now. Look at what I just shared. That 'me versus them' thing is a sure symptom of a hopeless perspective, as well as a clueless point of view. I'm embarrassed I ever believed the organization focused any attention on battling with me. I did not understand what was valued by an organization, yet I expected them to know and respond to my needs somehow."

Elli read the confusion on her friend's face and went about explaining it another way. "Too often I used to feel like a leaf in the wind at work. I depended on the winds of luck to carry me to the right places and keep me out of harm's way. I placed myself at the mercy of fate. I felt powerless to  have any real influence over my destiny. Even though my work was always important to me, I didn't know how to discover my work needs, much less how to satisfy them. I was lost, though at the time I didn't realize how lost I was. I let things happen and accepted that as the way it is. I can honestly say that there's no way I'd have my role today at work if it were not for RP."

"Now this may be relevant. That's the way I've been feeling lately. And now the hammer's coming down on me, out of nowhere." Cynthia was becoming even more attentive.

"Well, maybe not out of nowhere," Elli carefully remarked.

After a moment of thought, as if insulted, Cynthia suddenly charged like a bull. "Here's what I believe—work is a game of luck and chance. It seems that it's not what you know. It's who you know! If you don't have the right connections, you enter play by throwing well-formatted resumes at job descriptions, postings or classifieds. At no time are you informed about the constant changing of expectations, not in the job listings nor during the interviews. You stand by and wait to see whether or not you hit the target based on someone else's judgment. This person, by the way, very often does not know the job themselves. If you hit that target, in their opinion, they bring you on board. You do the best you can every day with inadequate information and infrequent communications while navigating shifting moods, constant changes, social politics and hidden traps. The game continues. Once a year, someone using a mandatory form announces how well you're hitting the supposed target. But that was yesterday's target, and the new target, if you know it at all, is only a moving, nebulous outline cloaked in fog."

Elli nodded with a caring smile, recalling how similar this perspective was to the one she used to hold herself.

Cynthia was now in a passionate rant. "Rarely does anyone ever sincerely ask you about what motivates you, what you can do or offer, listen to your ideas or care about how you're really doing or what you need from your work. You're just told you have to do more with much less, while finding new ways of doing it faster … and by the way, don't forget to be at all the meetings on time and pay attention to product quality, customer service, investors and ROI. You hang in there and keep at it, day by day, trying to dodge the layoff bullets and outsourcing missiles that might have your name arbitrarily inscribed on one."

Then she added with much more than a hint of bitter sarcasm, "We have employee satisfaction surveys so someone can place a check mark on his or her list, compile statistics, make reports and place them in a big file cabinet or database somewhere. Who says they don't care?"

Then Cynthia had another thought as Elli continued to nod periodically. "I hear we finally have a sincere conversation during exit interviews. That is, once you've decided you've had enough and are heading out the door for greener grass somewhere else, which, of course, is seldom 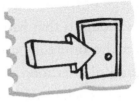 greener; rather it's just déjà vu with new names. Or maybe in my case, I'll experience the sincerity while being asked to pack up my things and being directed to the door. Then again, maybe I'll have to wait until I get to the outplacement counselor for anyone to be interested in what I have to say or what I want."

Cynthia was surprised that she had all these feelings within her. She knew her eyes were watery. She realized she was angry, actually angry. Or was she scared? Either way, what was the source of these strong emotions?

Elli wanted to get the conversation onto a positive track. She did not want Cynthia remaining in this state of anger and despair. There was no reason for that, even if Cynthia did not yet realize it.

On second thought, Elli realized Cynthia's venting could be healthy and constructive considering the intensity and nature of the moment. Getting disabling points of view into the open might provide new space in Cynthia's mind for more constructive thinking. Elli now knew how damaging and limiting toxic and unconstructive points of view could be. She also appreciated they could be hard to purge unless they were brought to the surface and acknowledged. She used to hold similar ones and had resisted letting go of them. Elli decided it was OK to let the poisonous thoughts that had been building for so long in Cynthia's mind become fully exposed to light and fresh air on this beautiful afternoon. After all, she thought to herself, if the disease is acknowledged, there might be receptivity for a cure. An eastern philosopher once imparted, "You have to drain a full vessel enough to be able to put anything into it."

Elli probed, "Is that it, or is there more to your perspectives about work?"

Cynthia reignited, as if Elli hadn't even spoken, "You know what's even more nuts?"

Elli followed patiently, chin in hand, "Maybe not. Share please."

"You never know anything about the forces or the logic that drives all of the crazy workplace stuff. It's just a great mystery. Why is there never any real candid conversation or authentic, substantive dialog that happens between hiring and firing? Sure you get orders and instructions, but it's so one-way. They just tell you what to do, and you respond submissively with a salute and OK, when or how? Asking 'why' is seldom acceptable or even answerable. The last time anyone seemed to listen to what I had to say was at my job interview. It's just nuts. If you're fortunate enough to climb the ladder a few rungs and gain the privilege of looking behind the curtain, you find only more curtains."

Cynthia rolled on, "From what I can see from my lonely perch, managers, supervisors and leaders are struggling too. They don't know why it is this way either. They're just running on their own treadmills, each trying the best they can to stay out of harm's way and make sense of it all, while still trying to project confidence and instill trust. The worst of the bunch put their heads deep into warm comforting sand. Sure, there are some outstanding leaders and supervisors. But that's why they're outstanding, they stand out from the norm! We notice them because they're an exception! Great supervisors should be the norm. Don't you expect every doctor, teacher, pilot or accountant to be a reliable expert in their job? Why is this not true for supervisors and leaders in the workplace?"

Silence again. Elli let the noxious thoughts ripple out into the open space of the coffee shop.

Then after a pause, Elli eased in cautiously, "Wow, until I listened to your thoughts, I forgot how I used to feel. Girl, you have some serious pent up energy about this stuff. No wonder I used to rage against the machine! You're right Cynthia. The way this stuff typically goes down at work is not in anyone's best interest … not the workers, not the supervisors, not the leaders and not the organization. Like gurus predicted hundreds of years ago and are still writing about today, workers and management are stressed to the max, anxiety-ridden, alienated or disenfranchised. Straight, honest talk seldom happens at work, and it's replaced by BS. Mistrust, confusion and doubts fester out of sight on both sides in everyone's hearts and minds. Rightfully so. Still the beat goes on, every day, and it does so in small and large organizations and within every profession and across every industry."

"Amen! You nailed it girl! The beat goes on!" Cynthia affirmed.

"Except, that is, where RP is being applied." Elli then added, "Cynthia, there are causes for everything, including all that happens at work. If you seek to learn the underlying causes, you can create dependable solutions and unlimited possibilities. RP begins with helping you know, discover or diagnose root causes to get the effects you desire and deserve. Even though you don't appreciate it at the moment, you have bountiful choices. Not realizing the source of personal power at work is the biggest obstacle to most workers' personal satisfaction. Often workers mistakenly believe the only way to make work more enjoyable or more rewarding is by leaving their organization. We resign ourselves far too easily to accepting the way things are. Every day, we go to

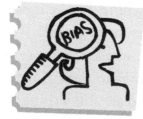

work with our heads full of opinions, assumptions, prejudices and bias. These have been formed by friends, peers, parents and media. Yes, many times they have been validated by our own experiences. But these points of view are inadequate, incorrect or incomplete. Some are toxic because they limit, confuse, disable, endanger or paralyze us.

"Work's a very big part of adult life. For many of us, we trade more waking hours of precious life and talents for work than anything else. Work's too important to not master it. It just makes sense to get smarter and become better equipped. The key to having security and attractive choices in our work is understanding the many forces in the workplace, both those forces in ourselves as well as those of our organizations. After all, *when work's good, life's better.*"

"And when work's not so good, life suffers," Cynthia said with confidence.

"On that, we can both agree!" Elli affirmed.

Cynthia then shared openly, "I admit, I'm not feeling confident that I understand work, what my boss thinks and needs, or even what I want from my work lately. My experience maybe hasn't helped as much as I thought. In fact, you're now implying it may actually be a disadvantage."

"Well, I would not go that far, but we do get programmed by the influences surrounding us. Enjoying far better communication with supervision is a key part of RP. Both workers and organizations get tangled up in interactions that seem like some strange form of socialized or institutionalized passive-aggressive behavior. There's typically politeness and friendliness on the surface, but there can be dark undercurrents, half-truths and information spinning which propel the words and behaviors on both sides. Both parties actually under-inform each other. This makes for a daunting puzzle that is unconstructive and harmful to both parties. Lack of understanding and dysfunctional communications hide the opportunities and choices both parties always have available to them."

Cynthia responded, "I think I can see what you're getting at. What workers and organizations say to each other and what they really feel are often actually two different things. In fact, communication is often pretty strange, if it exists at all. I know what I say to you or Dale about my work, but what I say to Rick is different, limited and, as you say, spun. It's the same situation, but totally different words. I bet there are similar things that go on when you compare what Rick says to me directly, and what he is actually thinking or what he says about me to other supervisors. I wish I could just be upfront with Rick like you and I are talking right now. And I wish I could know what he really needs from me and what he feels about me and my work as well. That would be so good. But I am not sure what I really want and need lately from my work. I think I've changed. But I suppose this confusion and these habits can be hard to break free from since they are deep-seated."

Elli encouraged, "Not as hard as you might think once you understand more about RP."

"OK, you mentioned hidden possibilities and choices. I'm not seeing that I have many options right now. I could use some possibilities and choices." Cynthia was more energized.

No matter how far you have gone down the wrong
road, turn back.
— Turkish proverb

How can I show you unless you first empty your cup?
— Nan-In

The first problem for all of us, men and women, is not
to learn, but to unlearn.
— Gloria Steinem

FOUR

SEEKING BIG AHAS

*Man's mind stretched to a new idea never goes back to
its original dimensions.*
— Oliver Wendell Holmes

With many of Cynthia's toxic points of view now exposed, Elli dug in deeper. "There's a bit of hidden irony here. You achieve your possibilities and choices by being the best choice and offering the most possibilities for your organization. If it's true that they may be thinking about letting you go, they would only do so if they do not believe that you offer them the greatest value from the options they have. By providing precisely what an organization desires, you gain awesome career leverage and power. Though simple and obvious, knowing how to do so has been surprisingly unknown. In part, this is because organizations are motivated differently than workers and no one has ever shared the secret with us. Also, seldom do organizations ever express their true needs accurately, completely or in a way that you understand. Here's where it becomes critical to have some 'Big Ahas!'"

"Big Ahas?" Cynthia did her funny face smirk, her head cocked sideways.

It had been a while since Elli had seen that. She smiled.

"Yep, a Big Aha is a term we use at work to describe a personal revelation. It's when you suddenly see everything in a totally new way. Once you have 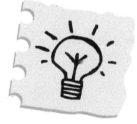 a Big Aha, things become so crystal clear that old ways of thinking are just pushed out, like a poison from your body. It's a 'eureka!' moment, you know, like your brain discovering a gold nugget. I've gotten a number of Big Ahas because of RP. I'll never look at work or myself in the old way again."

"Would it be possible to get a few of those Big Ahas right now? I need help tonight. Tomorrow will probably be a make or break day for me."

"I'm not sure we can get to them all, but we can try to at least get to a few this afternoon. It'll take a little time. There's a lot to cover, and I wasn't prepared to be a teacher or counselor today," Elli cautioned.

"You're doing great, and I'm game if you are," Cynthia responded hopefully.

"OK," Elli said. "Let's give it a shot. Now, as I just mentioned, workers and organizations are very different kinds of creatures. Far more than we typically realize. We're not talking apples and oranges here; it's more like apples and nails, totally different. Each party is pursuing very different objectives. Each is naturally acting in their own self-interest. Unfortunately, this self-centered focus tends to prevent both the worker and the organization from seeing what motivates and engages the very party they are trying to understand—each other. But again, there's this huge irony: each will better gain what they seek by accurately offering what the other seeks. This is so weird because neither has any natural interest in appreciating, knowing and giving attention to the other's needs, but interestingly, that's where the gold resides. The treasure has been hidden right in front of both parties all the time."

Cynthia pushed back, "Are you sure about this? I'm told what to do by Rick, and Rick knows I want to get paid well."

"So you're saying that you really know what Rick wants from you, right?"

"No, I guess not," Cynthia replied.

"And all you want from your work is to be paid well? That's why you've been so unhappy lately, right?"

"No, I guess not." Cynthia appreciated the ridiculous nature of her original comment.

"In a workplace, neither workers nor supervisors typically have complete and trustworthy information about each other's needs. Worse, each party doesn't usually understand their own needs very well! Worse still, each is different and self-interested. And yet, both try to form and sustain a lasting relationship with each other. Now, that's what I call nuts!"

"Relationship Performance may be more important than I realized, but I'm still a little skeptical," Cynthia interjected, becoming more fully engaged. She reached into her purse for a small note pad and pen. She began making notes. "Why are the organization's differences not more visible?"

Elli answered, "They are highly visible, if we know where to look. However, these differences are generally not seen because of our many filters. One of these filters is a result of the organization representing itself through the words and actions of its select people or representatives, such as supervisors, leaders, recruiters and so forth. An organization is a legal construct having a distinct charter. It is formed for serving a specific purpose or mission.

"Unlike workers, an organization does not have emotions, social needs or a life outside of itself such as family and friends. It does not speak directly, but through others who are placed into certain representative roles. When leaders, supervisors or recruiters try to express what the organization needs they often fail to do so completely. They are often only attending to a limited topic, situation or a subset of the bigger picture. In most cases, they, too, have never been told of the organizational perspective in an accurate manner. This condition also tricks us into believing we are interacting with other people who think and are motivated like we are. Actually, we are not. As workers, we are normally so focused on our own agendas that we have little time, attention or interest in trying to gain a better understanding of the greater organizational needs."

"This could get complicated," Cynthia murmured to herself.

Elli continued, "Not as complicated as you might now be thinking. But we do have to unlearn, then relearn. I guess this is a little like believing in a flat earth, and then discovering the earth is actually a sphere. You are just more aware of the realities you actually have."

"A Big Aha, in other words?" Cynthia smiled.

"Yes. Every organization has common, universal areas of attention that every worker should know and understand. Because we and our organizations are so different, when there is not full understanding of each other, it breeds antagonism and promotes confusion, dangerous assumptions, tensions or adversarial viewpoints. Each party can seem disconnected, uncaring, insensitive, disengaged, arrogant or indifferent. I now know that neither workers nor organizations are bad or ill intentioned, at least for the most part. We are simply and completely different and this causes misunderstanding. We have both been lost by focusing upon our respective needs and self-interest. Sadly this does not actually serve our self-interest since this thinking is not the best way to assure that we will get what we need. Understanding and leveraging the differences are the fountainheads of choice and possibilities."

Cynthia queried, "If we are so different, how will we ever be able to understand each other?"

Elli responded with good energy, "That's where RP comes into play. It's a practical and relatively easy way for both parties to know and think better about the differences, express needs to each other, gain understanding, then do what's needed to assure each gets what they're seeking. Each applies the RP organizing principles, raising the bar higher in their communication. Then they validate their understanding by agreement. Remember, *the only way for either party to dependably and consistently get what they need from the other is to provide what the other needs, and do it consistently with precision.* Choice is far more important for

agreement than you may realize, for having choices is one of the key factors that each must have in place to ensure that their needs are heard, respected and well attended. Both parties will continue to have a severe bias to their own self interest. Choice counterbalances these forces. *Choice is power at work.*"

Elli then became more intense. "Think about the implications of what I am saying. It significantly benefits the organization to know and be attentive to what you need, what you offer and what you think. This is the only way they can generate and sustain top performance from you each day or sustain a relationship with you, for you have other choices. Likewise, it benefits you in numerous ways to completely appreciate and be responsive to the organization's needs. This not only causes them to respond to your reasonable needs but also motivates them to keep you at the top of their list of choices.

"You win in both contexts, and so does the organization." Elli zoned in even more precisely, "Both parties must be extremely attentive and committed in order for either to enjoy the benefits. Awareness of each other's alternative options creates better attention and responsiveness. *Either party's indifference or restraint in effectively responding to the other's needs brings harm and loss to both parties.* My bet is, this relates directly to your situation with Rick as well as your recent personal dissatisfaction with your career."

"You may be right. But this is way too obvious. Anyhow, differences are always challenging, aren't they?" Cynthia was still hanging back a bit, reflectively in thought.

Elli nudged forward again. "Yes, that can be especially true when differences are cloaked in mystery, misunderstanding or dangerous assumptions. However, differences are fine as long as we understand each other and communicate effectively. But when we don't acknowledge differences, it is inevitable that strange, crazy and sometimes bad things will happen. In fact, RP reveals that it's actually wonderful and preferable that we and organizations are so different.

Because of our different needs, it's possible for both workers and organizations to get what they each want. This kind of partnership exists throughout nature. It is called a *symbiotic relationship*. Different entities get what they each need from the other while providing benefit to each other."

"I remember that from biology. It's like the microorganisms that are inside of us that help with our digestion. They help us, we help them, even though we each are totally different and have different but complementary needs." Cynthia recalled.

"Yep, that's an excellent example. Other symbiotic relationships include honeybees and flowers, sharks and remora, and fungi and tree roots. For that matter, trees and humans also fit this category. We exchange oxygen and carbon dioxide with each other by being very different. Both give and gain. It works perfectly. This is a big point, for in RP, it's imperative that you get the Big Aha in that *work should be symbiotic*. Both must benefit so each can reliably gain what they seek in a durable manner. *Work's a we thing!* RP caused me to understand that there is no competition between the organization and us, as we are sometimes led to believe. We can't buy into the 'us-versus-them' battles with each other any longer. Each party must attentively care for the other's well-being. There's no place for apathy, indifference, complacency or, worse still, antagonism or acrimony. We're all truly in this together. This is not soft, fuzzy-wuzzy stuff but hard facts."

"I've got the Big Aha! It really does cause you to see things in a whole new way, doesn't it?" Cynthia exclaimed.

Elli was pleased, "Yes, there's just no other way to have sustainable results any longer in today's workplace. Both get what they want by giving what the other wants. To do this, you use the rules and tools of RP—think constructively, have healthy dialog with each other, make sure your work role relationship is based on a clear agreement, perform well and keep choices ever present."

"Agreement again?"

"Yes, that's perhaps the most critical part of RP. At the center of good work is a complete and reliable agreement between the worker and the organization. It's just the op-posite of what you said earlier that you believed. You cannot leave any-thing to luck, fate or chance. Agree-ment provides for validation, clarity of understanding and balanced attention to each party's needs. It defines the  expectations and obligations in both directions, and up-front! It divides and distributes responsibilities. It elimi-nates confusion and assumptions. It is the map of the work relationship. Agreement always takes place in advance of work performance, not after the fact. Agreement serves as each party's guide or blueprint for their relationship. Sure, it has to be remodeled occasionally, but you always work in agreement." Elli had been careful to emphasize *in advance of.*

"This still sounds way too obvious, but it does sound possible." Cynthia was enthusiastic.

"Well, it is simple. Keep in mind though, that you have to each truly know what you need, understand each other's needs, set aside the time for healthy dialog and reach agreement. All this takes patience, empathy and negotiation. You cannot negotiate effectively without realizing that each party has other choices and options available to them. You also can't form a good agreement unless you are sharing complete and accurate information with each other. This encompasses what you each are willing to offer to the work relationship and what you desire to get from the work relationship. As you can anticipate, this type of dialog takes thoughtful preparation. And this agreement must be kept up to date, in both directions. Just common sense, right?"

"This seems to be the right way to work. It does seem to be just common sense. Is it too idealistic?" Cynthia still was taken aback by how straightforward RP was.

"I appreciate where you are coming from. I recall thinking that RP was blatantly obvious. But isn't that always the way it is with important breakthroughs? I also recall wondering why everyone was not already doing things this way at work. I don't have any good answer for why things are not this way everywhere. I only know that RP is a better way and it works. RP's radically different from the regular ways of thinking about work. And it's anything but idealistic. In some ways, it's just the opposite. It's much more realistic and practical than the way things have been done in the past. You could say that work that's still being done the old way is too idealistic, or perhaps said another way—naive; thus, it rarely lives up to our expectations. We must become more realistic, practical and personally accountable in accomplishing what we seek."

"That brings it home!" Cynthia affirmed her appreciation of the last point that Elli made.

"It does. The key is forming agreement and doing so at the front end. For example, depending on the retrospective annual performance review is like driving through the rear view mirror," Elli said, to make the point even stronger.

"And even then, looking at that rear view mirror only once a year!" Cynthia added.

"Right! Accidents would be inevitable and constantly occurring. And that's what's happening every day in workplaces. Without agreement, it's inevitable that suboptimal or dysfunctional things will happen. In most organizations without RP, even where there is sophisticated information and systems in place, such as one-way instructions, training, procedures, policies and processes, there's still no agreement. And as you might expect, the relationships are weak and fragile at best, or they often break. When they do fail, one or both of the parties scratch their head afterwards, wondering what happened, often with ill feelings toward the other. Then they tend to repeat the whole thing over again with someone else. There are just too many assumptions and too much ignorance present in most workplace relationships. Agreements done well and diligently assure complete understanding and prevent assumptions and inappropriate expectations. An agreement is the only dependable structure for a work role relationship." Elli emphasized *only* with a bit of intentional drama.

She went on, "In fact, often neither party even understands that to get what they want, they must first form, and then sustain, a strong, durable relationship. This is called a work role relationship. Sometimes the parties resist even trying to have a good relationship. They prefer to believe that work is an adversarial model instead of a cooperative one. When's the last time you've heard the word relationship in the context of your work?"

"Never," Cynthia said as if on cue.

"That's what I anticipated of course. Typically, some kind of affiliation is just assumed to be in place. Too often, both parties mistakenly believe they are entitled to their affiliation. There are many signs that this is true if you just look for them. Neither typically understands that a work relationship must be carefully formed, earned and nurtured. A work role relationship cannot just be assumed by anyone, ever. You know about the consequences of assuming, right?"

"Yep. Makes 'one' out of both parties." Plenty of relevance was appearing now to Cynthia.

"As we've already seen this afternoon, there are many anemic, incorrect, unconstructive or even toxic points of view in the minds of both workers and supervisors. It feeds on itself. In some situations, it gets real ugly, as you well know. Remember what happened at my Dad's company?"

"Yeh, I had forgotten about that," Cynthia recalled, shaking her head.

Elli was staying on track, "Remember your rant from only a few minutes ago? Both parties too often believe they are entitled to their affiliation. You clearly felt entitled in your work relationship and to be treated better. *With RP, there is no entitlement for either party.* Instead, both parties gain and sustain a work role relationship *by accurately offering the performance the other party needs.* In fact, how can it be otherwise?"

"Let me guess. That's why it's called Relationship Performance?"

"Sharp! Now you're tracking!" Elli congratulated.

> *God changes not what is in people, until they change*
> *what is within themselves.*
> — The Koran

"Well, I guess what you're saying is true and it may be a much better way of looking at work. But I have to admit, RP feels a little less comfortable than imagining I am entitled to something, even though I may not deserve it. With shared accountability, you're placing a lot of new responsibility on me, the worker. And I was so happy in my blissful ignorance and denial," Cynthia kidded, then she got serious again. "Do I simply sit down with Rick and talk?"

Elli continued, "Yes and no. You have to know what to talk about. RP is not just about talking. Plenty of talking is already going on between the two of you. RP is about sharing critical information that both parties must have and know. You need structure and you need to use a common language. By this I mean that you use frameworks, semantics and a tool called *rpWeaver*™ for guiding dialog. RP provides each of you with frameworks. You can think of these like maps for better understanding. Technically, these are just shared organizing principles to get everyone on the same page. RP also provides the process, rules, structure and tools so that you both dependably get better rewards. Notice that RP does this for both parties, not just one or the other. That way both parties are incentivized to apply it and stay with it. It's the only thing I've ever seen that is truly *neutral and unbiased*. It does not impose values on either. It helps both and favors neither."

Cynthia rolled her eyes. The message of doubt was clear. She was still not buying that fact about neutrality. Old points of view were resurfacing.

"Really!" Elli defended, "Don't worry, RP's not more  management propaganda or the employee motivation program de jour. In fact, RP introduces the concept that lasting work role performance is always a two-way street. That is, both parties must precisely provide what they have agreed upon in order to dependably get what they require and deserve. *Each party performing in a manner so that they remain the other party's best choice is the powerful force that holds a work role relationship together.* When you think about it, how can you skew or bias that? Furthermore, each party in RP must share responsibilities to achieve their two way-performance."

Elli continued, "If you take it seriously, RP makes work relationships that last, are enjoyable and provide both parties with predictable results. RP helps the worker or candidate just as much as it helps the manager or supervisor. It turns on a bright light so that everyone can see the realities of work and work relationships. It's liberating and empowering for both. It places both parties on an even footing to gain what they deserve."

Cynthia interrupted, "It sure is a radically different way of seeing things. Doesn't this pose a direct challenge to the status quo and conventions that many organizations hold so dear?"

> *The mind precedes all things, the mind dominates all things, the mind creates all things.*
> — The Buddha

Elli cautioned, "Yes, it can be a big change at organizations that want to stay put and cling to the old ways, keep people in the dark and resist the new realities emerging all around them. Even the most positive and rewarding change can be very difficult in most organizations, but most must now respond to workers with better methods. They must soon rise to the occasion, or their survival is threatened. Often, a change management program is applied simultaneously to RP deployment. In any case, if only the worker knows and understands RP, they become vastly more competent in navigating their career. But as you learn more, I think you'll agree that in the future, you'll only want to be at organizations that apply RP."

"Sounds scary but still realistic. Tell me more!"

Elli continued in a tempered tone, "Don't get me wrong, Cynthia. I'm not claiming RP is magic, a miracle or elixir. It demands personal thought, accountability, homework, assertiveness and attention. But anyone can use and enjoy it, if they try. I can tell you that I've seen over and over that it provides incredibly fast rewards and a path to major improvements for anyone who applies it and does so consistently. It might help if you think of it as a 'career fitness plan.'"

Cynthia was filled with new thoughts.

Elli recalled that Cynthia had always been an excellent student and a very fast learner.

Cynthia perused her notes then questioned, "What's this 'work role relationship' thing you've been referring to—a fancy word for 'job?'"

FIVE

THE END OF JOBS

We can't solve problems by using the same kind of
thinking we used when we created them.
— Albert Einstein

lli was in full-blown instructor mode. Coinciden-
tally, training functions were recently added to her
work role largely because she found deep enjoyment
instructing others. Since adopting RP, she and her company
leveraged her personal enjoyment because it amplified her
performance. Elli was pleased with how engaged Cynthia
was. This wasn't as hard as she envisioned a half hour ago.

Elli began, "There's a huge difference between a 'work
role' and the old term 'job.' The old concept of a job
doesn't serve a useful purpose any longer in progressive or-

ganizations. As a means of information, it's too limited and leaves too much unaddressed or not considered. In today's workplace, 'job-thinking' is too one-sided, inflexible and out of touch with the present realities of a growing number of organizations, workers and candidates."

"OK, go on." Cynthia felt something very important had just been said, though she was still in a fog of learning.

"Jobs, as we have thought about them and described them, are fodder for assumptions, false hopes and perpetual doubt. They leave everyone in the workplace guessing. As we've already touched upon, the cornerstone of today's successful workplace is a healthy *relationship* between a qualified person and their organization. Though a work role belongs to the organization by definition, a durable relationship with a person always resides at its center. Job-based models of thinking by either workers or organizations fail to fully structure and offer guidance to a healthy workplace relationship."

Elli continued, "Achieving a strong work role relationship is the responsibility of both parties and is accomplished by thoughtful design, discussion and understanding. It's not done by accident or wishes for good fortune and especially not by a shallow document like a job description. *A work role is a blueprint for achieving mutually beneficial work rewards for both workers and organizations. It's a better way of thinking about work and work relations.*

"Unlike a job, a work role's structure includes comprehensive and realistic information as to the organization's

46

functional needs and circumstances, specifications for a qualified, capable person *and* what such a person will need from the organization to be satisfied and to perform at their best. A work role's structure encompasses *both* organizational and personal requirements for a predictably rewarding relationship. A well-constructed work role instructs the supervisor, the worker, the recruiter and the candidate in how to form and sustain work relationships to provide everyone with the yields they seek."

"You're saying a work role specifically addresses the needs of both parties in the workplace, not just the organization's?" Cynthia questioned.

"Yes, work role information covers personal fulfillment and what the qualified worker or candidate requires from the organization to perform their functions in an optimal manner. But work roles also encompass and provide more information about the organization's needs as well. Work roles are based upon desirable organizational yields, or the ultimate purpose or reason for the work to be done, and the functions to be performed. Work roles describe the organizational responsibilities for personal functional performance, since RP is realistic in the premise that both parties have obligations in achieving desirable performance. Well-designed work roles include collaboration with workers to be assured that the relationship is equally rewarding and is validated to be lasting, or durable, for both parties."

"Are you crazy? In collaboration with the worker? You're kidding, right?" Cynthia wasn't quite as skeptical as she sounded. She instantly found collaboration in work responsibilities to be a radical, yet extremely attractive, concept.

"No, I'm not kidding," Elli smiled broadly. "The worker today must have a 'voice.' What's even more interesting is that their 'voice' is very valuable to the organization. Deep and fundamental changes have been taking place in the workplace over the last 20 years or so. We all intuitively sense that something big is taking place as we try to manage our careers. However, most of us don't quite know what to do, how to respond at a personal level, or for that matter, at a management or leadership level."

> *When any relationship is characterized by difference,*
> *particularly a disparity in power, there remains a*
> *tendency to model it on the parent-child-relationship.*
> — Mary Catherine Bateson

Elli went on, "Organizations used to be paternal and rather dominating. They made commands and demands then expected salutes and compliance. Typically, personal contributions were compensated with only a financial and benefits package. As they did so, they often provided implicit or explicit assurances of lifelong employment, if that's what a worker chose. Most provided a high degree of security to a worker throughout their lifetime, even into retirement years, such as with pensions and other forms of generous major lifetime benefit packages. Layoffs, if they happened at all, were temporary and lasted only a few weeks to adjust production output, change assembly line fixtures and so forth."

"That model was before my time," Cynthia said with a wink.

"True, that was our parents' workplace. Now increasing global competition, more demanding and finicky consumers and the upward ratcheting expectations of cold-hearted investors or Wall Street analysts will not let organizations operate in that model anymore. No organization can promise security or offer lifetime scenarios for a worker's career. The world is just changing too fast, and reality is too severe for that way of thinking."

"Yeh, I guess that's right, even though I sometimes forget all those factors. I wish things were simpler and not so seemingly vicious." Cynthia was filled with thoughts as she offered her words almost in a whisper.

"We all tend to forget the many forces that are impacting, influencing and driving organizational decisions. But all of our wishing for a simpler time will not change the present realities," Elli responded. "There's another big factor, or you might say, another side of the coin. Workers used to be like loyal patriots within those relatively stable and lifelong jobs offered by those paternal companies. Not only has the organization changed but so has the worker. Today's workers are more educated and informed. Many are also more conscientiously managing their careers to fit better into a fuller, well-lived life.

"Today's workers seem to be less puritanical workaholics and seek more 'balance' in all aspects of life, especially work. We, as workers, are more aware, discerning and mobile. It used to be that workers stayed with their organization through 'thick and thin.' It was actually seen as a negative not to stick it out, hang on and blindly entrust your career and work security to your organization's management, no matter what. Today, most of us workers are far less loyal. Many of us know we must take charge of navigating our best career paths. Remember the derogatory term 'job-hopper?'"

"Haven't heard that one in a long time! When you and I entered the workplace after school, it was a fairly common term, wasn't it?" Cynthia asked rhetorically. She continued, "No one wanted to be seen as a 'job hopper' on their resume. I really hadn't noticed this has disappeared. Hmmm, that's interesting!"

Elli nodded in agreement, "It's because it's not relevant anymore. You could say it's more quid pro quo, or something is only given for something that is gained, equally, in both directions. But, even now as both workers and organizations are more discerning, and with each having abundant options, they must also become even more vigilant in responding accurately to the other's needs. The success and survival of both parties are intertwined. The forces are felt in both directions and these pressures are greater than ever on everyone."

"And so are the anxieties, confusion and stresses. I feel them!" Cynthia exclaimed from a visceral level of personal experience.

"That's true. As we agreed earlier, now it's all about performance. Both parties must perform for each other's needs and do so with accuracy. It's a free market of talent where everyone has to be competitive to play and win. Assumptions, complacency and ignorance can be very dangerous. Organizations only seek and care for the best, brightest and most qualified people to be their most vital ingredient for thriving in today's economy. Both parties have to work together to dependably realize two-way, or reciprocal, performance. High quality communications are vital, as is the degree of compelling value one party offers to the other. Against such a two-sided, dynamic backdrop, it just makes sense that work is now collaborative. *Work's a we thing!* As you now can see, the way most people and organizations used to think about jobs is way too anemic, rigid and one-sided to address modern realities in the workplace. Do you also recall how people would sometimes remark 'that's not my job?'"

"Yep, I confess to saying that myself a long time ago, though usually under my breath. But I haven't thought that so much lately. In fact, I don't have any idea what my job even is anymore, and haven't known for quite a while, now that I think about it. It seems to change everyday," Cynthia recalled, as if she was speaking quietly to herself instead of to Elli.

"Constant change is a reality now. Can you imagine an admired and valued player on almost any winning sports team saying 'that's not my job?'" Elli challenged.

"Now that you put it that way, I guess not."

"That's because sports and a few other professions, such as acting, music, art and so forth, are designed for achieving top performance within a role. Everyone jumps in to offer what they can to win. Conversely, jobs are about minimum performance done consistently."

"Minimum performance?" Cynthia was clearly caught off guard by that thought. That didn't sound right.

"A little history might help."

"Oh no, a history lesson too?" Cynthia said, only half-joking.

"It won't be too painful. It's relevant and will only take a minute. This relates to the way jobs have been defined. 'Job' and the related term 'employment' are from the old days of the industrial revolution. That was when people were *employed* to run the machines of industry, literally and figuratively. The machines and physical infrastructure made

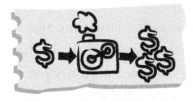

money and were central to both success and survival. Capitalism, including the means and the equipment of production, was key to building wealth, as opposed to people.

"Whether on the assembly line at Ford, feeding Eli Whitney's cotton gin or later on the line in a textile plant of just a few years ago, people were 'replaceable commodities' applied as *labor* to perform specific, repetitive and intentionally limiting jobs. People were just like other *resources,* procured and plugged into the company's assembly line, processes, construction site, procedures or operating consoles. They were analogous to fuel or supplies, hence the term 'human resources.'"

Elli went on, "It's important to note that in a job, achieving peak human performance or realizing the full potential of a worker was rarely the goal. Furthermore, personal fulfillment had little relevance to an organization, though it might accidentally happen. People were selected and used for a set of discrete skills to do certain functions in pace with the machines, processes or procedures. Those paced, structured, and limited activities were called 'jobs.' Whether people used for the jobs were called human resources, hired hands, employees, personnel or just plain old labor, they were not valued as investments but rather another operating expense or cost.

"In many cases, people in jobs were seen as a temporary solution, or a necessary evil, until a better, cheaper automated solution could be found or invented. People were disposable and exchangeable, even more than the parts of a machine in some situations. So you can see, in that mode, the organization's objective of employment was aimed at achieving only a minimum acceptable threshold of specific human performance offered in a consistent, reliable manner. Yes, work is still modeled this way by some organizations as well as by some workers. It's still the basic construct of job descriptions and performance reviews in some workplaces. But the world of work is now changing in deep and fundamental ways."

"I have never thought of any of this before, but it all makes sense now that you point it out," Cynthia responded, reflecting on her recent observations about her work, as well as Dale's "job."

Elli nodded and rolled on, "Today, in the best and most progressive organizations, the way work is modeled is completely reversed. The greatest wealth is being derived directly from people's potential, not capital equipment. In these organizations, unleashing the potential of people is seen as essential for the organization to thrive. A workforce like this is respected in new ways and described as 'talent.' Workers are seen as an *investment*, not an expense. By the way, that's one primary difference between talent and labor.

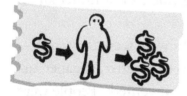 Talent is regarded as the vital money-making, competitive and innovative advantage in operations and strategies. People's performance, responsiveness, problem solving and creativity are valued as critical ingredients for success. Labor has jobs. Talent has roles.

"As I shared before, roles depend on solid relationships. Forming and sustaining durable relationships between the organization and qualified workers has become paramount. This is more and more evident at top national and global organizations. It's equally seen at the most successful local hospitals, car dealerships, schools, engineering, accounting or law firms and even neighborhood coffee shops, surviving manufacturers, services firms and call centers.

"People are now envisioned as talent investments," Elli continued. "And like an investment, they're being sought after to realize a maximum return on the investment, or ROI. Workers are being more precisely targeted and selected for capabilities related to *predictably* providing maximum performance in the work role. Yes, work is also now more unstructured and more loosely defined. The workers who have the highest value are the ones who are more autonomous and self-directed, who can accept change and be held responsible for doing the right things, in the best ways, in a variety of situations. The concept of employment has flipped. It's interesting to me that everything being reversed means organizations now *employ* technologies, infrastructure and other capital assets to facilitate and amplify people's performance. That's just the opposite of the labor model where people were employed to get the performance from the machine or assembly process."

"Sort of a strange way of putting it, but I see what you mean," Cynthia responded. Then she offered, as an example to test her understanding, "In my situation, computer software is 'employed' by the company to help me think and perform better."

"Correct!" Elli affirmed. "This fundamental change is not really strange when you consider the pressure that most organizations are under nowadays. Most of them reached a point of diminishing returns with the labor model in the latter part of the last century. People who were employed in the labor model were generally used for what some call their 'below the neck' abilities, such as using their backs, arms, legs, fingers and hands. Most jobs were very physical in nature. Organizations now have to constantly figure out ways 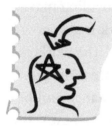 to do things better or to even totally reinvent what they do. Unleashing the power of people above the neck, that is, capitalizing on the worker's fully engaged mind, including intellect, knowledge, experience, judgment and creativity, is now the objective. Peter Drucker, one of the foremost management gurus of the last century, long ago predicted this change as the rise of the 'knowledge worker.'"

"Never saw my neck as 'the great divide!'" Cynthia laughed as she said this.

"I love using that to make the point!" Elli said. "So you see, a talent model of work is now used for creating *maximum* performance and productivity as organizational investments. This includes the constant harvesting of new ideas, new ways of thinking about existing problems and the discovering of new opportunities. Innovation is now a clear expectation in almost any work role. The suggestion box is no longer a place for chewing gum wrappers that are never gathered.

"The talent model changes everything. To recruit the right workers and to achieve their maximum performance, work roles must be designed to offer more than only money and benefits, since peak personal performance perfectly parallels personal fulfillment and enjoyment in one's work.

"Prior reliance on 'command and control' mechanisms of management no longer provides the responsiveness and flexibility that organizations need for competitive and innovative advantage. Leadership, management and decision-making today are more distributed throughout the organization into all of its communities and reach all the way out to touch and engage every associate or worker. The best organizations are applying both hierarchies and human networks to their advantage, and again, they are doing so by design."

"What's the difference?" asked Cynthia.

"Hierarchies are based upon *authority*, as designed and assigned by the organization. On the other hand, networks are based on the *trust* that emerges organically as people communicate and work together. Every organization has both in place, but in the past, only hierarchies had been acknowledged and respected for gaining productivity, such as the use of org charts, reporting structures, chain of command, etc.

Organizations now realize that networks can powerfully propel or hinder their progress. Think about it ... how much actually gets done in your organization by networks versus the official chain of command or 'org chart?'"

"Well, I'd say that in our case, almost everything gets done by networks!" Cynthia exclaimed. "In fact, look at how I found out about the mess I'm in. For example, Gerald is definitely one of my go-to guys in my workplace network. Without the network's magic, we'd be at an operational standstill in only hours. We are constantly swinging on our network grapevines to overcome the shortcomings of our organizational structure."

"Exactly, and that's the way work works. In truth, both hierarchies and networks serve distinct and important purposes. One engages when the other fails. So as you might expect, they typically oscillate back and forth, though

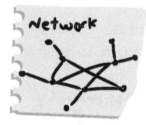

we seldom notice this dynamic taking place. One more related point—a hierarchy is confined to the organizational census since it works only by authority and thus only within its walls. On the other hand, human networks have no limitations, so they extend outside of the organization's authority boundaries, even into other organizations and personal networks.

"In fact, look at how you and I are connected to each other professionally and how our relationship can potentially impact both of our organizations, such as you now being trained by me today in RP's basics. Networks are even more important when you have a talent model. Networks are a means to gain optimal performance from talent and to find new talent, by leveraging the power of professional and personal social interactions. Remember, networks extend far beyond the walls of the organization."

"The talent model is a really big deal, isn't it?" Cynthia seemed on the cusp of having another Big Aha.

"It really is, Cynthia. It's a paradigm shift impacting everyone who works. Modern automation, robotics and a variety of technologies have displaced much of the need for labor and jobs in more and more workplace situations.

"Furthermore, outsourcing entities around the globe now have numerous advantages when it comes to exploiting the labor and jobs model, especially in the cost control area. This is particularly true now as time and location boundaries disappear," Elli added.

"And many other countries have a far greater supply of low cost labor to fill jobs!" Cynthia was clearly paying attention.

"For sure! Even local fast food drive-thru and newspaper writing jobs have been staffed by people on the other side of the planet."

"You're kidding me!"

"No, really! But the talent model is a whole new game. Organizations and workers are together becoming what you might think of as 'creative hives,'" Elli said smiling.

"Creative hives? So I'm back to being a worker bee again?" Cynthia didn't see that one coming.

"Not in the way you think, but interestingly, perhaps much like in the way bees actually perform their roles in nature. Workers now must be constantly learning, performing and innovating. Workplace gurus advise that *each worker must be a lifelong learner and offer self-reliant personal leadership to their role* in order for organizations, as well as themselves, to survive and thrive. They can't depend on all the answers or specific, complete directions being handed to them. They must perform their role by problem solving and making good decisions, often independently. To make the creative hive work there must be effective communications and actions that are focused on what is good for the community. Actual beehives seem to be successful in a very similar manner."

"Oh boy, I have had so much so wrong for so long. But in my case, ignorance certainly has not been bliss." Cynthia was shaking her head back and forth slowly.

"Well, we're taking care of that now. I see you might be having another Big Aha about the talent model's impact on the workplace." Elli offered the words both as statement and question.

"I think I am! I have been frustrated recently because I haven't been told exactly what to do by others, but you're causing me to see that I share accountability for this. I must be part of the answer. I also see that our organization must get into the talent model and do so soon!"

"Precisely, friend! That's now a part of your work role and you have to rise to the occasion. The talent model brings a new level of expectations for the worker, but it also offers new possibilities. People who are considered talent at work are chosen to play their part in roles much like top athletes or actors. I'm sure you appreciate this as another good reason for the name work 'role.' And just like acting, the role has to be designed and the right actor cast so that it works optimally for the producer and director's screenplay. In your case, the screenplay is the organization's mission and strategies. Equally, the actor's needs must be fully satisfied, or in your case, the worker's or candidate's. It's normal for roles to be constantly modified, evolved, shifted and changed. Unlike jobs, sometimes work roles can be quite nebulous, thus much is often left up to the qualified worker to figure out."

"I think I get it, Elli. I kinda like seeing myself as talent." Cynthia smiled, her chin held high. "But the talent thing is not totally new, is it? I don't just mean in Hollywood, modeling agencies, orchestras and pro-athletic teams. Haven't some workers been thought of as talent before now?"

"Yep, you're right again. There have been a select few, such as those folks in top management ranks, or sometimes stars in a sales force, who have been considered and treated as talent. This has been true even when the rest of the organization was considered to be labor. Talent models apply to others such as some seasoned, successful attorneys, scientists, professors, consultants and doctors. In such cases, those people were seldom seen to be in limited, minimum performance jobs. They had roles where both maximum performance and self-directedness were expected. You can be sure both parties' needs were served, including by forming and sustaining a strong, durable relationship.

"On the other hand, it's also true that many other professionals in the past, such as nurses, engineers and teachers, have been considered as just another form of labor placed into jobs. Yes, even an organization's management and leadership have been, and still can be, categorized as either talent or labor. There's no rhyme or reason to this, but the implications are significant. In fact, this still varies incredibly from organization to organization, and it sometimes varies by industry and profession. But the workplace is generally shifting from labor and job models to talent and role models, due to more gain and less risk. This major shift, in part, explains why there are new kinds of unrest, confusion, tension and anxiety in workers, supervisors and leaders. It also often explains the root causes of both successes and failures in companies and institutions you may read about in the business section of the news. At a personal level, this shift certainly puts a whole new slant on career planning. *To be safe and to succeed at work today, a person should ensure they are seen as highly valued talent, rather than as disposable labor.*"

Cynthia jumped in, "Whoa, this is a really big deal! It is now even clearer to me that we are still in the old world of jobs and labor in my workplace, and I think I am beginning to see why some things are not going so well with us lately, or with me for that matter. We've lost a lot of clients, we're on the verge of losing others and our profits are pretty razor thin. We've also lost a lot of very good people. Maybe the folks who left were actually talent, but we were treating them as labor?"

"Perhaps, but if that's the case, you can quickly correct this with RP," said Elli. "Remember, jobs were one-sided. There are two *sides* to a work role. The two perspectives address the many separate personal and organizational dimensions that are a part of modern work. Great people, like you and me, are now perhaps the most important investment an organization makes. Or more correctly stated, we should offer the personal value to an organization so that we are thought of in that way. We must *earn* a new level of respect and power. Conversely, we must be provided attentive *stewardship* if our personal potential is to be fully unleashed. It only makes sense that smart organizations should be doing everything they can to gain our full potential. You know what's very cool? If our potential is fully unleashed by strong *Talent Stewardship*™, we are happier in our work as we simultaneously perform better. It's a real and practical win-win situation."

"Amen to that concept, sister!" Cynthia blurted out in response to Elli's sudden combination of motivational speech and old fashioned sermon. "What's up with this 'stewardship' stuff? Sounds like labor union jargon."

"Interesting that you should think that. In fact, in the old labor and jobs model, often the only recourse workers had for advocacy and attention to their personal needs were labor unions. Remember, a job was one-way and since the organization only sought minimal performance, attending to personal needs was of little relevance or benefit to them once the minimum performance threshold was being met reliably and consistently. Hence, labor unions filled the vacuum and predictably used the term 'steward.' Stewardship is one of the best words to describe providing accurate attention to workers' more comprehensive needs. But also note, they're called labor unions." Elli emphasized the term "labor."

She continued, "In a talent model of workforce investment, a smart organization should be well-motivated, due to its many incentives and reasons, to provide attention to personal needs. Such attention leads to a new form of *balance* in the workplace. They respond to workers' needs in order to better serve their own needs. Doing so is to their distinct advantage and is like caretaking for any other investment. It's very risky not to do so. In fact, they must do so to competitively attract and keep the highest quality of workers. So the organization must provide thoughtful and well-designed stewardship to both workers and candidates. This just means being more responsive to workers' needs to assure that those needs will be met. Again, this is another reason for the two-sided term 'work role.'

"As you might expect, in RP you'll hear talent stewardship used often. Talent Stewards in an organization practicing RP will be people you have known as supervisors, managers or recruiters. In other cases, it may be a person in an entirely new role established to address the growing needs of workers, candidates and work role design. *Talent Stewards serve as 'brokers of performance' since they attend to, and serve as advocates for, the needs of both the organization and those of the worker or candidate.* With talent, focused attention to people and two-way performance cannot be relegated only to the traditional HR department. Nor will one-size-fits-all approaches work any longer. Each work role will be unique. And the workers within each role will have unique differences that must be attended to in order to successfully form and sustain relationships."

"Now that makes a lot of sense." Cynthia remained attentive, but also quite reflective.

"It does, doesn't it?" Elli then added, "And by the way, you may be hearing new terms bandied about lately in business journals, books and so forth. These validate something big is changing in the workplace, though not yet fully understood. These may be weird, nonsensical terms that use old words in new ways, like they're now calling workers 'human assets' or 'human capital.' But beware of dangers related to these casual terms. Even though talent is an investment, it cannot be an asset, since talent is comprised of people. Assets and capital are owned, people are not.

"There is rightful possession and entitlement to assets and capital. On the other hand, people have discretion and free will. We exercise choices every day, in all kinds of ways. We choose to enter into a work role and we can choose to leave it. Assets don't have brains to think or legs to go where they desire. We people do. We go home at night and choose to come to work the next day, by choice. People are not owned, thus cannot be considered as assets or capital. The reason I emphasize this is that the words we use, or don't use, are important. Words not only communicate, but they also serve to shape or reinforce points of view, for better or worse. Terms like *human capital, human assets* and, one could even argue, *talent management*, tend to sidestep the importance of work role collaboration and shared work role relationship accountability. Assets are owned; however, talent works by mutual attraction. So again, *work's a we thing* for today's best workers at today's best companies."

Elli then concluded this point with emphasis, "*RP clearly is based upon the premise that neither party has entitlement to a work role relationship.* Both parties have to constantly merit and earn their work role relationships by being

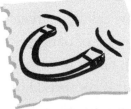

the most attractive option that the other party has. Continually offering value to each other is just like creating a powerful magnetic force between two objects."

Cynthia jumped in, "Wow, I've never thought of work even close to this way. I could see if the value is not there, there's no magnetism. In fact, you could easily and unintentionally repel the other party in some situations if you are only working on assumptions!"

"You've got it!" Elli congratulated.

Cynthia added more, "Though, now, as you enlighten me, I realize that I've always had some form of disdain for the word 'job,' and especially for thinking about myself as only an 'employee.' I've wanted to be more than just a cog in the machine. I've always wanted to be considered as more than just a human resource. I have also wanted to know what my role in the company was really worth or how it was valued. There's so much more that I can offer, especially if I am in the right work role! By the way, now that you mention it, lately they've been calling the workers 'human capital' in our organization's newsletter. Isn't that interesting?"

Elli continued, "Well, perhaps we can consider that as positive at this early stage. At least it indicates someone's waking up to the big changes that are underway. They may not have it all figured out yet, but you and RP can help them get there. At least they don't think of workers as labor, a resource or worse still, a 'necessary evil' any longer."

They laughed together.

Then Cynthia frowned, "Well, that may not be true about me anymore."

"Just hang on and stick with me, girl," Elli encouraged. She sensed that Cynthia had anxiety about tomorrow morning's uncertainties.

"RP is utilized by organizations to unleash the power of people, and to do so by design. They apply RP in their own self-interest to gain the yields they desire. By the way, putting RP into practice within an organization is called *Work Role Yields Management*™ or *WRYM*™.

"Everyone benefits with RP. People are sought after and stewarded as talent to be fully engaged and satisfied within their work roles so the organization can dependably gain the yields they seek. That's not just a play on words nor idealism, but a whole new perspective and a very pragmatic philosophy. RP enables both parties to be responsive to the changes that are underway in the workplace. RP begins with you, the worker. It does so by outfitting you with a better and more complete point of view as to work relations."

> *To know truly is to know by causes.*
> — Sir Francis Bacon

"This sounds empowering!" Cynthia had recovered.

"It really is, but you have to keep in mind that being seen as talent instead of as labor doesn't let the worker off the hook in any respect. RP means accountability for everyone. *In RP, workers appreciate that they must always be doing whatever they can to be the best investment and choice for an organization.* With RP, workers and candidates realize they must be more personally valuable and competitive in their workplace, and for that matter, in the greater talent marketplace of their chosen professions. Lifelong learning, top role performance, innovation and flexibility in response to changes are all basic requirements for workers and candidates today."

"Now that puts a damper on my viewpoint! It seems easier being labor and just having one of those 'good old jobs.' I can see that more is expected of talent within a work role. And just as I was beginning to relax and feel a little cocky." Cynthia conveyed learning in her dry, tongue-in-cheek style of sarcastic kidding.

"Sure, jobs are easier for those who want only to offer minimum performance doing the same thing, day in, day out. But is that really who you are and can you afford to take that risk any longer? Keep in mind, if you're seen as only labor in today's workplaces, it's hard to find a safe place. And no, as talent, you can't afford to be arrogant or have any sense of entitlement. Certainly not in RP! RP can make you pretty humble and sometimes a little paranoid, even though it takes place in a constructive, realistic and productive way. Remember, RP's called Relationship Performance for a reason. More importantly, RP only equips you to be able to understand the new world of work and to use that knowledge to get what you want and need for yourself."

Elli went deeper, "RP's neutral and balanced to mirror emerging workplace realities. RP provides both parties with the knowledge and tools they need to form and sustain healthy and durable work role relationships. It also provides

a common language so that they can communicate more pro-
ductively, for until now there have been problems even in
the language used between workers and organizations. This
has created confusion and misunderstandings."

> *One ought not to be thrown into confusion*
> *By a plain statement of relationship ...*
> — Robert Frost

"Got that for sure! Sometimes it seems as if good
communication is impossible with Rick when he's in supervisor mode. Ironically, I can easily speak with him anytime
as a friend about non-work stuff. It's sort of weird actually."
Cynthia said this in an emphatic, but also reflective and diagnostic tone.

"That's not weird. It's normal, unfortunately. But it's
also no longer acceptable, for it presents both personal and
organizational risks. A common language that's practical
and usable for effective communications is imperative. And
the language must be based upon dependable, shared principles about the way the world of work works, including
how to appreciate each other's needs. This may be the most
important part of RP, though it may be hard for you to envision at the moment. Better communication causes both
parties to have better thinking and understanding, which
usually results in better empathy, perspective and actions
within their work role relationship."

"That was a mouthful. You sound like a real expert, Elli," Cynthia offered as a compliment.

"I have to admit, I take this very seriously. Doing so pays me dividends every day, not only at work, but also in many other parts of my life which are directly and indirectly affected by my work. RP has become a 'career operating system' for me. Thanks to RP, I've gotten the challenging assignments and promotions I wanted; I've played a part in shaping my own work role around my life's needs. More importantly, I'm happier!"

"I'm beginning to see how RP could be very good for me as well. I also see that work roles and work role relationships might be a big and complicated topic." Cynthia was trying to keep up. She felt as if Elli's words were coming at her like gushing water streaming full blast from a fire hose. She had a lot of gaps in understanding that needed to be filled. She was writing furiously.

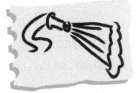

"They can be," Elli affirmed. "Work roles are unlimited conceptually, though each one always tends to have a distinct 'center of attention.' Work roles can be designed to be general or specific, limited or expansive—whatever is needed to provide the organization and the worker the rewards they are seeking. They are based on crafting clear instruction, specifications, agreement, guidance, measurements and support, not just for the workers or candidates, but also for others who steward the work role, such as supervisors and recruiters as well. This information can be relatively straightforward and brief, or very complex. Most prefer to do this within a process of continuous improvement and continual refinement across time. But what's best, however you approach work roles, is that they are not constrained by the anemic, one-way information, breeding misunderstandings, with old job-type thinking."

"Like our job descriptions?"

"Precisely!" Elli said, "How much does your job description pertain to what you were actually doing today?"

"Not at all! Zero! Zilch! In fact, our job descriptions are totally out of date and irrelevant to what we actually are asked to do each day. They're a joke. No one uses them, except maybe someone in HR for regulations or whatever."

"That's often the case. Most work changes too quickly now for traditional types of static job information. Your organization needs for you to more broadly understand their needs and to appreciate their expectations of you in a more complete, expansive and instructive way. This includes bringing your attention and creativity to possibilities and problems that no one would envision within a job description. The organization needs similar information from you about your life requirements and career desires. Work roles are more complete by design. A work role is a blueprint of how we, as talent, connect to and relate with the organization. Remember, in RP, this connection or affiliation is always done through a special form of relationship called a work role relationship.

"To ensure that a work role relationship is correct, valid and acceptable to both parties, there must be agreement. In today's world, a situation where either party is operating on assumptions regarding their work role relationship is fraught with potential problems. That's why I'm so emphatic about the word 'agreement.' It is essential for work role relationships. *Agreements are the only way relationships can be reliable for either party.* And work role relationships are at the center of how both parties get the yields and rewards they seek from the work that is done."

"And based on what you're saying, I can now see why performance reviews are out of touch with today's realities. They are for jobs!" Cynthia interjected.

Elli replied enthusiastically, "Absolutely, and brilliant of you to say so! Performance reviews are often based on the concept of jobs. Worse still, they are *after the fact, quite arbitrary and often based on out-of-date minimum performance models.* By the time you get them, too much time has passed, or you might say, they are too few and far between. Sometimes they arrive too late for effective performance remedies or repairs of relations. Like jobs-related thinking, they are normally only one-way, 'pointing the finger' at the worker as to sole accountability for performance. Yesterday's performance reviews were not constructed on the full set of applicable organizing principles that address shared performance accountability. Performance reviews are generally another component of an increasingly obsolete employment model that was a part of labor and jobs. Like

I shared before, they are like driving forward by looking through the rearview mirror.

"Can you imagine a winning sports team, orchestra or the cast of a movie depending on annual reviews? Of course not! They offer their expectations and feedback up front and continually. Then they perform to that agreed-upon criteria every day. In fact, those folks do this much like what is done in RP. They discuss and agree as to how performance will be defined in both directions, then get into agreement about what *each will be offering* for that performance and how they will *measure* it. Then they both work to stay in agreement. Feedback is provided regularly to ensure both parties that they are staying on track for the other."

Elli continued, "In RP, you occasionally may have 'agreement reviews' as either party needs. RP is two-way performance by design. RP agreement is up front and with constant attention versus one-way performance reviews, which are occasional, retrospective and sometimes almost forced and arbitrary. I like to think of RP agreements as a 'will be' for both parties while performance reviews are a 'was' or a 'could have been' or a 'should have been' for only one party. It's no surprise that labor and jobs thinking naturally led to the 'us-versus-them' points of view!"

"This really makes sense! I am beginning to see the many dimensions you are referring to when you say *work's a we thing*," Cynthia said smiling, while still making plenty of notes.

"It also makes for a greater probability of happiness and success in our work." Elli was smiling as well. Teaching others was always satisfying to Elli, but sharing these ideas with a friend in need was extremely gratifying.

Elli once more reinforced some of the points so they were firmly anchored in Cynthia's mind. "So, as you can see, the word 'job' and even 'employee,' as it refers to a person, are relics of the past. That is, unless you are in an organization that is still operating in the past. Work now must be right for both parties, and both parties must work together effectively to make it right for each of them. I realize I took you on a long trip to deliver these points, but knowing the big picture should become a big benefit to you. But there may be something you didn't notice in what I said that you find even more interesting about the shift to work roles."

"What was that?" Cynthia was truly enthusiastic and curious.

> *An invasion of armies can be resisted, but not an idea*
> *whose time has come.*
> — Victor Hugo

SIX

REVOLUTION

Elli continued teaching, "By the very nature of a work role, *both parties* are accountable for the performance of every function that exists within a role. Think about the implications of this." Then Elli intentionally paused.

Cynthia reflected on that point.

After a few moments Elli resumed, "That is radical for most workplaces, even though it's just more common sense. For a variety of reasons, organizations have not accepted their own responsibilities for a worker's functional performance. Instead, explicitly or implicitly, they have held the worker solely responsible for the performance of his or her functions. Again, RP's philosophy is more connected to reality. Capable talent must be well utilized by the right environment of support, outfitting and enablement in a manner conducive to optimal performance. RP enlightens everyone to the fact that there can be no optimal role performance unless both parties are doing what they should be doing to make that performance happen consistently. In other words, with jobs, work was a 'you' thing. With work roles and RP, in yet another context, *work's a we thing.*"

"Now that has the makings of a revolution!" Cynthia declared. "If I understand you correctly, I would not be held solely accountable for performance in my work functions. Each party would have responsibilities for the performance of each function. In other words, the finger would not be pointing only at me!" Cynthia's expressions were revealing the enthusiasm of newfound knowledge.

"That's exactly right. As to revolution, it's only a revolution for the workplace because we've been so primitive. Both share credit for the good and both share accountability for the bad. Look at the credits at the end of a movie. Why do you think they call them credits? It takes everyone to make a great movie, and producers and all who are a part of the production realize this. It certainly takes a lot more than only the leading actors, no matter how good they are. And to get the best from even the greatest actors, it takes great direction, supporting casts, stunt people, set design, costumes, editing, lighting, logistics and so forth. Even my hubby knows when he's coaching the middle school basketball team that it takes the staff, the school, the plays and strategies, the parents and all the players acting in purposeful harmony, as a team and by design, to have a winning season."

Elli continued, "Another example would be the elementary school classroom. It takes the student, teacher, setting, curriculum, textbooks and parents to achieve consistent performance. Everyone must perform, not just the students. True functional performance within any organized environment is always more than one player acting alone."

"That's so true! I feel like I have capabilities, but I don't have the support system," exclaimed Cynthia.

I had been my whole life a bell, and never knew it
until the moment I was struck.
— Annie Dillard

"Of course, the worker must be capable. This includes being motivated, competent and attentive in doing their part in work role performance. But delivering performance also includes training, development, coaching and information. It is inclusive of reasons, instructions and feedback, facilitating infrastructure, tools, equipment, safety considerations and a long list of other environmental factors. A work role's design should offer a blueprint encompassing all of the respective performance factors of a work role relationship, not only the person's accountabilities, skills or prescribed actions.

"A work role includes both parties' obligations, needs and requirements for every function that should be performed within that role. Both parties provide what they must to generate optimal performance for each function of the role. This clearly is another reason for the merit of upfront agreement, so these shared responsibilities can be discussed, considered and determined."

"This redefines accountability, doesn't it?"

Elli went on, "Yes, it makes it more expansive, inclusive, collaborative and more closely aligned with how optimal performance is created and sustained. A work role finally addresses the fact that functional performance is always both parties' responsibility. Accountability for performance is distributed, more complete and more defined for everyone. Performance is not a burden that is unrealistically or exclusively placed upon the worker alone. In other words, for every function a person does, there are many things both parties must contribute in order to get the desired results. Each party has specific accountability, but that's what is so important ... that each have their own accountabilities."

"So the worker is still specifically accountable, yet both are accountable?" Cynthia appeared to be working out the details of this in her mind.

Make everything as simple as possible, but not simpler.
— Albert Einstein

"Certainly! *The worker must offer the capabilities, including the competencies, soft and hard skills, traits, qualities and sustainable motivations to perform the work role functions superbly in that environment, or possess the willingness to gain those capabilities. On the other hand, the organization has the responsibility to well utilize, steward, outfit and enable the worker's capabilities so they predictably achieve optimal performance together. The organization must also ensure there are not factors in place inhibiting performance, including mediocre peers and weak or toxic management and leadership. Greater diligence in talent selection is also important in RP.*

"An organization is only as good as its talent selections. Providing workers and candidates with literacy about RP, then equipping them to practice RP, is another example of organizational responsibility that leads to better functional performance. That's quite a bit different than the way your performance is judged presently as a 'you thing' in the old workplace."

"And is compensation a part of this?" asked Cynthia.

Elli nodded, "Ah, yes, compensation. In RP, compensation is seen in a more complete way, not only limited to money, financial incentives or benefits. Everything an organization offers to you in return for your personal performance is considered to be compensation. After all, if you look compensate up in 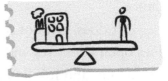 the dictionary you'll find it means 'to counterbalance.' So in RP, compensation includes money and benefits but goes far beyond that into any aspect of the work role that creates a satisfying work role experience.

"Compensation includes everything that counterbalances the value you provide to the organization. It involves extensive considerations of the satisfaction you must get from your work and related contexts of your life in order to have a durable work role relationship. Compensation also involves eliminating the factors that cause dissatisfaction in your work. We both know that money and benefits alone seldom provide lasting satisfaction at work."

Cynthia thoughtfully responded, almost with a degree of reluctance, "Well, though I've heard and resisted that fact before, I have to admit that's true. I've had great income and benefits, though I don't use many of the benefits. Even with these, I have been miserable at work lately. Does RP

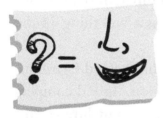 offer anything to guide you in discovering what it takes to be happier at work? Maybe I can use this information to help me make better decisions about what to do next, whether at my current workplace or even at another one. I'm starting to feel the power of choice."

"It does, but not so quick," Elli snapped back. "RP does open your eyes wide to what may provide happiness, satisfaction and fulfillment for you at work. It reveals causes of boredom, toxic stress, frustration and dissatisfaction, which are equally important. It provides tools to predict the

experience you will have in a work role, in advance of being in the role. However, *in RP, you can't pursue happiness in your work unless you first master work role security.* In other words, there can be no fulfillment in your work, unless you achieve work role security. *Having career choice begins with having career security.* Personal work role security is paramount for workers and candidates. How can you ever have the promise of satisfaction at work, if you don't have any security that you will be the chosen person to be in that role tomorrow?

"RP offers frameworks that guide the worker called *Work Role Mastery*™. This map helps you see and mentally organize a dependable basis for having *security, fulfillment* and the *realization* of what you seek and deserve from your work. You use this as a guide for seeking agreement, making better career decisions and marketing your value in a more effective way to your organization or to other organizations. You apply this basic knowledge for navigating the complicated landscape of work to find success and enjoyment. If you have the time, let's try to cover at least the basics before finishing this afternoon."

"Security put first? That's surprising. I think I could use some of that right now. More Big Ahas, if you please. I have the time," Cynthia said with a broad smile, while still making notes.

Inspiration may be the revelation of something completely new, but it is also the rediscovery of something always true.

— Robert Grudin

SEVEN

WORK ROLE SECURITY

> *It does not pay to leave a live dragon out of your*
> *calculations if you live near him.*
> — J.R.R. Tolkein

E lli reassured, "Cynthia, I'm sure you would have seen security as a first step in RP if you'd had the time to think a little about it. Look at the situation you found yourself in today. *Work role security has to be the foundation that your work fulfillment is built upon.* And just like the foundation for your house, a work role can be no better than its foundation. What good is it to be really happy in your work if whatever you're doing offers no assurances that it will be there tomorrow?

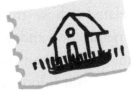

Many people who are terminated for whatever reason were happy until they sat down, unknowingly, in front of their boss' desk for the last time. If you don't first give attention to securing your work role relationship, you're always treading upon thin ice. And that thin ice tends to crack at the worst moments, and there you are."

"And there I am!" Cynthia agreed. "OK, I can accept that, but how can I make my work more secure? Do you have some kind of manual on this or something?"

"Your basic guide as a worker in RP is a reference manual called *Career Fulcrum*™. All of what I am sharing is from that one book. I'll see if I can get a copy for you," Elli responded.

"Thanks, but I mean fast, like in the next hour!" Cynthia was clearly motivated.

"OK, patience. We'll march through a few basics. Hang on." Elli felt like a drill sergeant right now. "By now, you get the point that a work role is a unique form of relationship. Especially the way I've been hammering in the point about that! It's certainly not like marriage, friendships, family or parenthood. Although, too often, we treat it like one of these other kinds of relationships, which can be a bad mistake. None of those are *solely* performance-based. Work roles are. Our security at work is directly related to how strong our work role relationship is with an organization and that is based on performance. And performance has many dimensions and contexts."

"But I don't really have control over that."

"That's what I used to think, but I was wrong. Both parties actually have a great degree of power. That is what leads each to having the options and possibilities that keep their work role healthy. In most cases, you will have more control over this than anyone else."

Elli took out her trusty pocket planner, tore out a blank page and with her pen, she began to draw on the torn paper. She drew two horizontal lines, one on top of the other. She labeled between them **Security**. Then Elli placed the words **Attraction** and **Agreement!** in circles at each end.

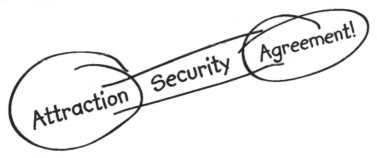

Cynthia was as eager as a fine thoroughbred horse in the starting gate while Elli was drawing. "Let me get this straight. To master my work role, I have to first think about work role security. And to have security, I have to create and manage a work role relationship with attraction and agreement?"

"You've got it, but there's much more. Work role relationships are held together by a combination of 'attraction' and 'agreement.' Both are equally essential. You can't be assured of having 'security' unless these two factors are in place at all times. They are the two pillars of a work role relationship. You also might consider these to be like those two tubes of chemicals that come in a package of epoxy glue. You mix these together and you have a strong glue. It's the same with attraction and agreement between a worker and an organization. You have to mix them together to create a strong, secure relationship that holds together. When both are in place, work roles are relatively secure, barring unforeseen circumstances and catastrophes. Keep in mind, nothing is risk-free and stuff can always happen that is unexpected. RP offers no promises or certainties, but it does cause work roles and careers to be much more reliable, predictive and probable. And no matter what happens, by applying *Work Role Mastery*™ you are better prepared and more resilient in whatever you need to do, or respond to, throughout your career."

"Can you explain attraction a little? I think I get the reasons for agreement. In fact, now that seems imperative in any work situation."

"OK," Elli responded. "To begin, attraction is what you offer to an organization that it values. *That it values* are the critical words here. Personal value is much more than just skills, competence, education and experience. Value includes the way you think and solve problems, the way you make a team better, your creativity, stability, dependability, energy level, attitude and engagement, your self-reliance, ideas, risks mitigation, responsiveness and resourcefulness.

All of these combine to comprise the valued personal capabilities you offer for the organization to utilize in a work role. Interestingly, your *relevant motivations* are always the single most important quality that smart organizations consider about your potential. Keep in mind, motivation can be situationally positive or negative, depending on what the organization needs or deems undesirable. And motivation, like enthusiasm, is an internal thing within each person. The right sustained motivations can overcome many obstacles. But no one makes or controls your motivations but you."

"Hmmm," Cynthia was reflective.

It is not enough to be busy, so are the ants. The question is what are we busy about?
— Henry David Thoreau

Elli went on, "So, all of these factors are a part of being attractive to an organization. Yes, performance and attraction are the same when considered holistically. And you've got to think about them in the way the organization thinks about them, which I'll describe to you in a few minutes. But first, let me reinforce some points. Attraction is a powerful force, like magnetism, that holds the relationship together. And just like magnetism, the wrong or conflicting capabilities, and especially the wrong motivations, will repel."

Cynthia understood, "This makes so much sense. In fact, now that you share it this way, it seems like I have to build and market my capabilities to an organization in a very effective way and do it all the time. So to be secure in my work role, I must be attractive to the organization. Again, common sense."

Elli affirmed, "True. It really is very similar to marketing because here is another rub: *attraction is always, and only, defined by the other party.* In the worker's case, this is the organization, or more specifically, their representatives such as supervisors, leaders, managers or recruiters. They are your 'buyer,' so to speak. Unfortunately, just like in other cases where someone is buying, often the buyer does not think well about or express their needs. That's why as the seller, you have to understand their needs as well or better than they do."

"So you are saying that I must know how the organization is thinking about my value even better than they do?" Cynthia questioned.

"Yes, that often is true. You must be the expert when it comes to the value of you within your work role. I think you'll see what I mean, especially when you consider that only you can best know *the product of you* and all the qualities and upside that you have to offer." Elli was aware that this could all get confusing at this point, but she knew that the *Work Role Mastery Framework*™ would make everything much clearer as she presented it step-by-step.

"One more reminder about attraction," Elli now had a cautious, serious tone in her voice. "Keep in mind that organizations have choices too and they are always looking for their best options. They have to do so. You must always be the most attractive option for a work role to ensure that your position is secure. This means you must be a better alternative than the worker down the hall, at the doorsteps or across the ocean in another country.

"Sometimes you are even being compared to an entirely different process, a new technology or maybe a company's sales rep that is promising an interesting miracle or silver bullet up in the executive suites, such as outsourcing your role to them. You've got to stay alert about being the most attractive option to your organization, since they always have their eyes open too.

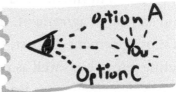

"Sometimes, this even means coming up with ideas to eliminate your own role completely. That's usually the most reliable way to get an even better role for yourself, even though it might sound counter-intuitive."

"My chest actually tightened as you said all that stuff. Sounds like a big new pile of stress and worries," Cynthia shared with a newly wrinkled brow.

Elli responded, "Not really. I'm only sharing the realities already taking place around you at work. You've been in ignorant bliss as you say. It's so much better when you know. Now you can be more vigilant in your work role and have your focus on the right things and act in the right ways. This makes for security. Remember, security is your solid foundation for getting what you want and need from your work. And another thing, if you have an agreement and are meeting the expectations it spells out and what you promised, you usually have little reason for constant worry. If you are not in agreement, as is the case with you and Rick presently, there is constant jeopardy for you, as you learned today."

> *... there is nothing more debasing than the work of those who do well what is not worth doing at all.*
> — Gore Vidal

Elli continued, "And this is another reason for seeking and staying in agreement. In fact, you can think of the process of agreement, in part, to be a little like personal marketing research, as well as personal salesmanship. As you pursue agreement, you learn what is wanted and you also can present your relevant qualities which may not have yet been known or considered. This really helps bring into the open what the organization defines as attractive or valuable. That's why I asked if you and Rick are in agreement when I first got here.

"You can't just go by your presumptions, nor can you rely on what you've been told before, even in documents or web sites. Agreement may bring to the surface what the organization doesn't value or may even detest. It allows you to present traits, experiences, knowledge and aspirations that the organization might not be aware that you offer, but needs. It can be really surprising how many false assumptions both parties can have if they don't seek and get agreement. It's the only way that you can confirm, or validate, that what you offer and what you are doing is indeed attractive to the organization. It's the only way the organization can learn the full value and potential of Cynthia."

"Wow, now that you share it that way, everything still seems so obvious. Even so, it seems like Relationship Performance is radical, as I said before, maybe even revolutionary, especially for our workplace. I could see this being like a rocket booster for one's career."

Elli realized she was being redundant but it was intentional, for it had even been hard for her to fully understand "the reality thing" in the beginning. "It can. It has for me. I'll keep saying this over and over, Cynthia. Relationship Performance helps us to better respond to the way the world works. We've been playing without the rule book, then wondering why we weren't winning. Unfortunately, many candidates or workers still don't fully know, accept or respond to the reality that surrounds them each day. Unfortunately, this is equally true for many supervisors, leaders, candidates and recruiters."

Then Elli tested to see if she was on track with Cynthia's needs this afternoon. She realized that she could get fanatical. "I realize today may not have been the best time for a classroom lecture. And I've probably drifted into an old fashioned sermon, but I thought maybe a little guidance and coaching might be helpful before you go back to work tomorrow. Do you mind if I take a bit of time to 'lecture' a little more?"

"Not at all. I'm hungry for help and now I appreciate why you are so enthusiastic about Relationship Performance. This is just what the doctor ordered for my meeting 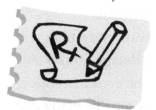 with Rick tomorrow." Cynthia was still fully engaged. "Do you mind if I first repeat back what I think I comprehend at this point to make sure I'm keeping up?"

"That would be wonderful!"

Cynthia then fed back what she had just heard with an amazing degree of clarity, only occasionally looking at her notes. "RP helps both parties form and keep lasting relationships with each other. This is based on each party having a shared knowledge and a common language to describe the way the world of work works. The worker and the organization come together in a work role to form a relationship, or more accurately, a work role relationship. Work roles are comprehensive blueprints that address both parties' needs, as well as their separate accountabilities. This approach serves to assure they get the results they each seek. Both parties apply reliable principles or frameworks to discover and accurately understand their needs. Then they share their respective needs and validate their understanding in a process of seeking agreement with each other. After reaching agreement, each simply meets their commitments, responsibilities and obligations to the other to get what they each have agreed upon. From time to time, either may need to change or modify their agreement because of inevitable things that may occur with either of them."

Cynthia then pointed to Elli's sketch that was lying on the table between them and went on. "A worker's first priority has to be establishing and keeping their work role relationship secure. If they do not have security in place, little else matters. They do this by making sure they are the most attractive option that the organization has for the work role and they validate their attractiveness by forming agreement. RP is basically imperative literacy for today's workplace that everyone must have to succeed."

"Wow! Incredible! An A+ performance! You've got all the makings of a Relationship Performance expert." Elli congratulated Cynthia.

"Well, I think right now I need to know a whole lot more about the organization's viewpoints and perspectives of attraction that you promised." Cynthia was a hungry student, which didn't really surprise Elli.

Elli was grinning as she called home to let her husband know that she would be later than expected. Cynthia knew Dale was working late on a project today, so she saw no need to call.

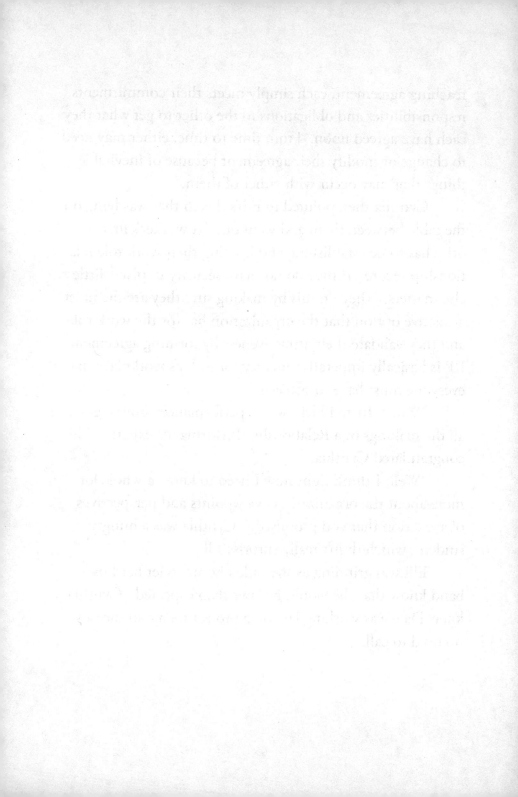

EIGHT

ATTRACTING ORGANIZATIONS

A fter getting off the phone, Elli began by referring to her drawing. "Now, let's talk more about the attraction aspects of Work Role Mastery. Either as a worker, or as a candidate, we always need to be confident that we are attractive to an organization. This is determined from the viewpoints of its pertinent representatives, such as your supervisor, recruiter and leadership. Remember that 'beauty is in the eye of the beholder.' We cannot be the judge of our own attractiveness. However, we can understand and be responsive to what makes up attraction. With that knowledge, we can be very smart and attentive to being and staying attractive. Attraction or performance falls into three distinct and different dimensions, even though only one is commonly known and described. We explain and understand these by using RP's *Organizational Triangle*™.

"We must apply the Organizational Triangle in seeking agreement to ensure we completely understand all the many contexts of attractiveness for our work role. In this respect, agreement provides the additional feedback needed to confirm we are on track with what is most attractive to our organization. You recall, with attraction and agreement in place, we have security. The practice of Work Role Mastery leaves little to doubt or assume."

"Organizational Triangle?" Cynthia queried.

Elli then started adding a triangular shape next to the word Attraction, talking as she quickly sketched. "Yes, every organization seeks and responds to people in a similar manner and does so in three distinct areas: Outcomes, Resources and Risks. *A person's value, or lack of value, resides in each of these areas, even if they do not know it.* These three dimensions of talent's value or appreciation are universal. They apply to every organization, to every worker and to every candidate. They apply to you right now at your organization. They are in Rick's mind, even if he does not realize it at the moment. In fact, these three factors form the basis for most organizational decisions and actions far beyond matters that are only about talent. This includes how it decides what to buy or not to buy, in what to invest and the thousands of other decisions made each day within organizations. It's not enough just to give attention to only one of these dimensions, for all three must be considered and acted

upon in order to be truly and reliably attractive to an organization. In Relationship Performance, these three important factors comprise the three corners of the Organizational
Triangle."

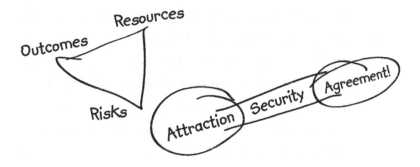

Elli finished the triangle she had just sketched by
scribbling three labels at each corner: **Outcomes, Resources**
and **Risks.** She explained, "The Organizational Triangle is
central to you being considered valuable in the workplace
and especially to being secure in your work. It defines
what's attractive, as well as what's unattractive, about a
worker or candidate from the organization's point of view.
As you might already suspect, the Organizational Triangle
offers a worker like you awesome leverage to get whatever
you seek and deserve throughout your career ... that is, if
you apply it and respond to it accurately and effectively.
Accordingly, it can reveal dangers by causing you to better see holes or gaps that may not have your attention, or
factors that may be missing in your assessment of personal

value at work. What's best, it can cause you to see a cornu-
copia of new opportunities for personal contributions that
will be valued and respected."

Cynthia studied them and said, "This is already so
obvious to me, yet it was so unknown! How's that possible?
I bet I might understand each of these. Just to make sure,
can you elaborate a bit on each of them?"

"Certainly! I warn you that there's more to them than
meets the eye at first glance or even that we will be able to
cover today. Outcomes is the most well-known corner of
the three. In fact, that can be a big problem. Sometimes
this is the only corner that is discussed even partially in the
workplace. ***Outcomes are what the worker produces, provides, creates, innovates and delivers each day in their
work role. This is the corner related to your personal productivity. Outcomes are the combined outputs from the
various functions of your work role.***"

"Is that the same as results, deliverables and return on
investment?"

"Generally speaking, yes. Outcomes include all that
the organization articulates or instructs that it requires in a
work role. But it can be much more since, in many cases,
many organizations do not consider or cannot imagine all
the potential a worker can offer, such as hidden and unknown qualities or aspirations, new ideas, new ways of helping their fellow workers, different approaches to problem
solving and so forth. So outcomes also include the many
potential values and qualities that a person can offer that

have not been specifically requested but perhaps would be valued and appreciated. Again, you validate if these qualities are valuable, or not, by using a process of dialog and agreement. Obviously, the more attractive outcomes a worker can offer, the more secure he or she will be in their work role relationship."

Discovery consists of seeing what everybody has seen,
and thinking what nobody has thought.
— Albert von Szent-Gyorgi

Elli added, "Interestingly, outcomes can be either positive or negative in the view of the organization. This is because a person may be feverishly producing outcomes, but they are not appreciated or valued since they are not what the organization actually needs. This is surprisingly common. Test question: Who is the only party that can define what is attractive as an outcome, or for that matter, what is attractive as it may relate to any part of the Organizational Triangle?"

Cynthia instantly responded with the correct answer, "Only the organization. I see that now, but I didn't see it before." Then she queried, "I suppose resources are what the organization provides to get and keep the worker, right?"

"Again, you are right. But again, resources from an organizational point of view go much further than most workers, or for that matter, many organizations appreciate. Resources include everything an organization should offer to get the performance they seek from a qualified worker. This is their side of the functional performance equation that we discussed earlier. It includes things like management attention, tools, equipment, facilities, training, compensation, safety, benefit packages and programs, development programs, coaching, mentoring and everything else that an organization must provide to seek and form relationships with qualified workers. Resources include all that they must do to attract and select the right candidates to join with them in the work role."

Elli continued, "Resources also include many different contexts of time; for in RP, time is typically one of the most precious resources. Time is considered in the context of productivity: how long it will take for the worker to become acceptably productive and how long the relationship will last. So you can see that providing outcomes is not enough; for to be secure, a worker must provide the greatest outcomes with the least possible resource demands on the organization. *The fewer resources that a worker requires, the more attractive they are to the organization, that is, outcomes being equal.*

"Even seemingly easy and insignificant actions can reduce resource demands that range from being more self-reliant, being prepared for meetings, making the extra effort to improve team dynamics and even bringing high quality new persons to your organization who are in your personal and professional networks so their recruiting expenses are reduced. All of these add to your value. On the other hand, workers requiring excessive management attention, who are not resourceful or who are inattentive learners, require extra resources. This makes them less attractive. *In your work role, the outcomes corner must be maximized and the resources corner minimized. Being an unreasonable 'resource hog' or 'resource burden' is a very serious personal liability."*

"This seemingly simple little Triangle could get complicated, couldn't it?"

"Work realities are more complicated than most of us realize. RP just helps us to understand this. Most of us have very little or no formal education in the things that matter most in life like parenting, marriage, personal finance or career management. RP at least gives us some help with the career management aspects of our lives."

"Well, at times I've felt pretty stupid in all four of those areas you just mentioned!" Cynthia laughed. It was good to see her normal, relaxed, smart and confident personality reappearing.

"Haven't we all? Now to the final corner: Risks. Organizations generally detest risks. They do whatever they can to minimize, mitigate or eliminate them. They realize that within any activities, there may be risks present. Thus they have a limited and modest degree of willingness to accept prudent risks, if they must, to get the gains or outcomes they seek. However, *a worker has a distinct advantage in their attractiveness if the organization envisions that the worker reduces risks by their presence in the work role.*

"Being a cause of errors, making mistakes, spreading discontent, not being innovative, not addressing problems quickly, causing disruptions in meetings, irritating customers or co-workers, being disorganized, having harmful or unsafe workplace practices, quality deficits, generating confusion, gossiping, being abusive to co-workers, poorly representing the organization in the community and not playing one's role well in teams are just a few examples of risks that some workers present. *Also, in this corner, the opposite can be true, because some roles require that the person be willing to take certain carefully managed risks to get the rewards the organization seeks.* Additionally, some workers are seen as more attractive, because their very presence, attention and traits are seen to eliminate or minimize risks and uncertainties. Again it all depends on the role, the worker and the organization's perspective regarding risks."

"Now that's powerful! All three are equally critical, aren't they? Let me repeat this back to you to see if I understand the Organizational Triangle correctly. To be truly attractive to the organization, the worker must concentrate their attention and perform well equally across three areas: *outcomes, resources* and *risks*. They must seek to optimize the outcomes, while keeping the resources burdens and risks to a minimum in their work role. *It's not enough just to be responsive to only one of these areas. Instead, you must be considering how you are, or are not, valuable in all three areas, all of the time.*"

"Precisely! And I especially like the fact that you understand you have to keep your eye on all three corners. If not, you will inevitably be blindsided. Each is equally important! You can be a great producer, be very self-reliant, be a risk watchdog, or you can be scurrying around doing what you think to be the right activities but still be in jeopardy because you are fatally off in one or two of the other corners."

Then Cynthia came to another Big Aha. "What's horrible is that I now realize I do not have adequate information about any one of these three areas in my role now. I am working in the dark and just hoping for the best each day. I know hardly anything about the outcomes corner in my role and 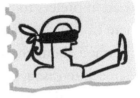 absolutely nothing about how the organization is thinking about me and my role in the resources or risks corner. That's really dangerous, isn't it?"

"Yes, it is," Elli affirmed. "This might explain why the rumor mill is abuzz about you. This is the situation with so many workers and their supervisors today. In fact, most are hired and then many are fired, laid off or outsourced without ever gaining this information that they so sorely needed to be secure and to succeed at work. And most candidates do not have a clue that the Organizational Triangle is the secret to gaining and keeping the role of their dreams."

Elli then went forward with her instruction, "Here's more guidance related to the Organizational Triangle. You should keep in mind that, as with almost any type of information that relates to understanding, you must consider what is called the positive and negative space or bias. It is just as important to know what is not wanted or valued as it is to know what is valued or wanted for each corner. In other words, it is important to know the *outcomes, resource demands* and *risks* that are both *undesirable* and *desirable*.

"You must look at both sides of the coin in order to have complete understanding. You should assume nothing. You should gain information as to the resources the organization prefers to extend or to offer as part of their investment in utilizing your qualities as well as becoming well-informed about those they prefer not to offer. You must also seek to discover the risks they actually desire or accept as a part of the role, along with those that are unacceptable. RP's Work Role Mastery demands that the worker or candidate becomes knowledgeable by learning both positive and negative information. You use the Organizational Triangle to respond to the organization's needs *with precision*. This allows you to apply your energy for being attractive without any diluting, wasting or jeopardizing energy being expended."

Elli continued, "The Organizational Triangle encompasses both strategic and tactical perspectives. Said another way, long-term and short-term views are taken into consideration. This would include what a person offers in their present work role or within a series of work roles in which they may advance. This depends on the nature of the role, but you can imagine that for most people, organizations may consider a person's value or attractiveness in one or both time frames. So should you. *Generally, it is best to think separately about what your value can be to each of the Organizational Triangle corners in the immediate, short term, tactical time frame as well as in the longer, strategic time frame.* This may include how you do, or do not, desire to advance into other work roles in your career. Often an organization may be looking at you as a long-term investment, and may be willing to take the long view as to their investments in you. If this is the case, you should know this."

"I get it. I've certainly never thought of my value to an organization in the tactical and strategic dimensions of time. This is humbling," Cynthia said while making more notes.

> *Humility provides everyone, even him who despairs in*
> *solitude, with the strongest relationship to his fellow*
> *man, and this immediately, though, of course, only in*
> *the case of complete and permanent humility.*
> — Franz Kafka

"Yes it is and personal humility is a very good sign," Elli affirmed. "In a way, you have to provide a degree of leadership as to what is possible in the work role, for many times you will see possibilities that the organization has not yet envisioned. But there's a little more that may be even more humbling to you. You now see that the organization is always viewing you as an investment for the value you offer in all three corners: outcomes, resources and risks. I continue to remind you that they are always looking at you in each of these areas in comparison to their other options and choices related to your work role and the yields they are seeking from it. You might say that all of us as workers or candidates have competitors in regard to all three corners of the Organizational Triangle. We generally know down deep this is true. Sometimes we don't like to think about it. But think and respond we must."

"Do you mean being compared to other co-workers?"

"Yes, but each of us as workers has many other competitors in our work role as well. Certainly you are being compared to co-workers. But also you are being compared to other candidates who are at the doorsteps, across the nation or even across oceans in other countries. Thus to be secure in your work role, you must always remain competitive and vigilant in making yourself the most preferred option that the organization has."

Elli went on, "Keep in mind, there may be available options you are being compared with such as outsourcing to contractors, automating by installing new technologies as well as breakthrough innovations that eliminate entire processes, methods, procedures, products or services related to your work role. It's not enough to just be vigilant about your work role. Look at the entire ecosystem that surrounds it to gain clues as to how you can add value. This is not good or bad. It's just a fact. Every organization must be competitive to survive and thrive in today's ever-changing world. You have to stay alert to how they act and respond to circumstances. The Organizational Triangle is key to having keen awareness about how organizations reach conclusions and make decisions about you and the value you offer compared to your competition, whatever or whoever it may be."

Cynthia commented, "So you are saying that organizations are not necessarily cold-hearted, mean-spirited, uncaring or insensitive. Instead, you are proposing that they are just pursuing their best options to survive and thrive? They are just 'decision-making engines' always trying to make the right decisions for success and preventing failure, however these are defined."

"Correct! Organizations are not people per se, though they are comprised, in part, of people and have people making decisions for them and being their voice, including investors, customers, vendors, boards of directors and so forth. Organizations typically serve a focused or a dedicated purpose. Often this is known as a charter or a mission. They are influenced and they are regulated. Most have severe pressures from many different communities simultaneously. Just as you and I choose the mutual funds we invest in, which are made up of organizations, we look for the best return, for the least investment with the least risks, right? How much do we care about anything else?"

"That example brings it home! This is all so true!"

"Very few organizations actually act maliciously or desire to cause intentional harm, although people within them can sometimes be guilty of human weaknesses, mistakes and malicious intent. Organizations simply strive to do what is best for the organization, its mission and the many constituents they must serve. They do this by constantly applying the Organizational Triangle to their decisions and actions. As the ancient adage goes, 'it pays to understand the ways of a dragon if you live near one.' When we work for an organization, it pays to understand its ways, how it acts and how it makes decisions. What's more, by understanding this, we can often get what we want in our career by being very attentive to providing the organization exactly what it's looking for. By doing so, we will be more secure in our work roles."

Cynthia remained attentive. "And you must perform, as a whole, or in each corner, better than the other options that the organization has or it would naturally and rightfully choose another option better than the one you offer. Have I got it?"

"Yes," said Elli. "You're a great student. I had no idea that I would be teaching tonight. I hope I am giving this subject justice for your needs."

"I am impressed! Why haven't you told me about this before?"

"I tried! Remember?"

"True, but this is really important! Everyone should know this. How can you survive in the jungle of work otherwise?"

Elli agreed, "I don't know how anyone can survive without this knowledge. People struggle with work just as organizations struggle with worker issues every day. It just doesn't have to be this way. But back to the topic, remember, no matter how well you understand the Organizational Triangle, or no matter how well you believe you are right on target in offering value to its needs, you never can be assured of this in the absence of agreement. To validate that what you offer to the organization is deemed as valuable to them and to fully understand what they really want from you each day, you MUST seek and form agreement with the organization. *Sometimes you have to have an agreement-related dialog before you even get a reasonable or complete understanding of the Organizational Triangle for your work role. Almost always you must inquire and not expect this information just to be handed to you on a platter. More often than not, it takes both parties to discover and fully see the work role relationship's possibilities. Hence, collaboration is an essential part of forming agreement.* This is typically done with the direct supervisor, manager or leader serving as Talent Steward for the work role relationship."

> *Can two walk together except they be agreed?*
>
> — Amos 3:3

"Will this be a written agreement?" Cynthia asked.

Elli was drawing a couple of stick figures, apparently shaking hands, in a very abstract manner to say the least, as she continued to instruct. "It does need to be documented. There should be certain measurable key indicators to ensure that there are no misunderstandings and that expectations are being met in both directions. Often the most important part of agreement is the prior preparation and structured dialog for understanding and preparing commitments that each party makes to the other. This is the heart of collaboration. RP has a tool that helps with this called *rpWeaver*™. This simple device helps both parties to prepare for dialog, then provides both with structure for the dialog so each can get their needs, values, requirements and qualities completely revealed and considered."

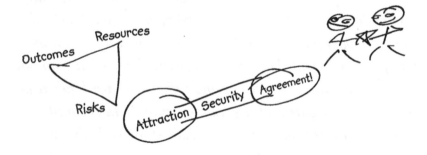

Elli explained further, "rpWeaver also provides a way for you to discuss respective expectations and to creatively negotiate in order to reach a point of mutual agreement. Afterward, you clearly know what is expected of you. You also have a process for how to meet any changing needs that might come up in the future. No assumptions, remember? The Organizational Triangle is one major part of rpWeaver's structure."

"What about my needs?" Cynthia asked.

"Good timing! That's the other part of rpWeaver's structure. Remember that RP brings what both parties need into a work role. Making sure that you are also satisfied is essential for your top performance as well as keeping you with the organization. So it's necessary that an organization be responsive to these factors, within reason, even if you do need to remind them from time to time." Elli smiled and rolled back her eyes.

"After all, how many athletes, musicians, engineers, accountants, nurses, upholsterers, salespeople, doctors, pilots, soldiers, police, truck drivers or mechanics do you know who are top performers who do not really enjoy what they are doing, who they are doing it with and the effects that doing their role has upon their life?"

"None, now that you put it that way." Cynthia suddenly seemed to be totally lost in introspection.

"Is anything wrong?" Elli asked. Was Cynthia daydreaming all of a sudden?

"No, not really. I think I've had a revelation about a number of things that may be very important to my situation! All of this seems so true, yet it seems alien and so different."

"Revelations are good I suppose, especially revelations about the realities of work. I guess RP often feels alien because so many of us have been flying by the seat of our pants most of our lives as to how we manage our careers! Analogously, the cockpit of a modern airliner, or even one of 50 years ago, would have seemed very alien to Orville and Wilbur Wright."

"Roger that … and as of this morning, I am in danger of a crash, without even knowing it."

"Perhaps you are just in a dive or a stall, since there's no crash yet. My bets are that there's still time for repair and renewal."

"I hope so." Cynthia's sincerity was evident.

Elli got back on track, "Back to what I was sharing. It is in the organization's best interest to do what it takes to assure that you are enjoying your role. This will motivate you to achieve consistent high results. In turn, your satisfaction will provide a strong incentive for you to stay. A smart organization understands that they have to be competitive to keep you with them. So now that we have described what the organization needs from your work role, we need to talk about what you need from your work role, right?"

"Right."

"So collaboration related to your needs is equally important to the strength and health of the work role relationship. But do you really know your own needs? Can you express them accurately and completely? They usually are related to your motivations, qualities, personality traits, preferences, aversions, desired rewards, desires and sense of purpose about the work you do. These make up how an organization will sustain a durable relationship with you. Factors in your work, the people you work with and many other aspects of your life have relevance, don't they? Got a little more time for your old friend, newfound teacher and career counselor?"

Cynthia's head had been nodding at the questions, then she stated, "Absolutely."

"OK, let's order a fresh cup of joe and some nibbles. I'm getting hungry. I teach. You buy this round. Deal?"

"Deal!"

In nature there are neither rewards or punishments,
there are consequences.

— Robert Ingersol

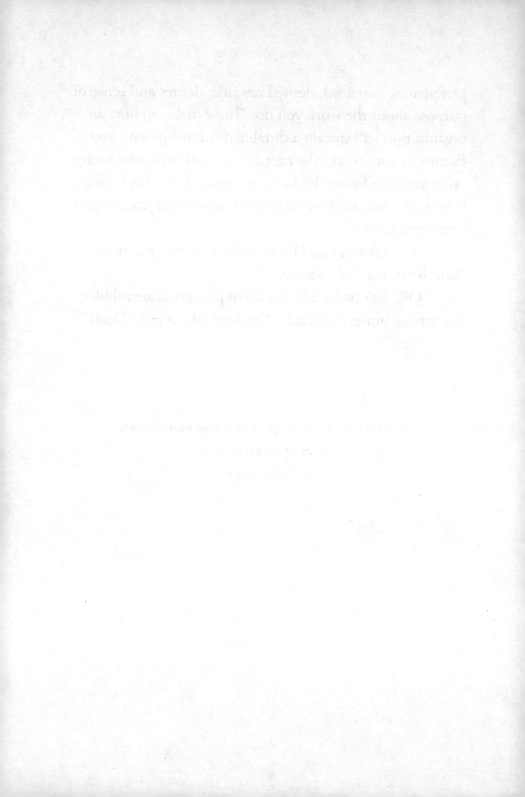

NINE

THE FULFILLING WORK ROLE EXPERIENCE

*Work joyfully and peacefully, knowing that the right
efforts inevitably bring about the right results.*
— James Allen

As beverages and plates of assorted munchies were brought to the table, Elli could tell that Cynthia was hungry for more than food. She had already filled many pages with notes. Elli's work role now included being a certified RP instructor for workers in her organization. It felt really good to be helping her friend.

Elli was drawing yet again. She was adding a new area below Security. "We each have a responsibility to navigate our best path to happiness, especially in our work. We can't expect others, including our organization, to do this for us. Satisfaction at work is vital to our overall happiness. In RP, this is called **Fulfillment**." As she said this, she was printing that word in a way similar to the way she had previously with Security. Then she added a couple more circles and words to the informal representation of RP's Work Role Mastery framing. Inside the two new circles she added the words **Are** and **Do.**

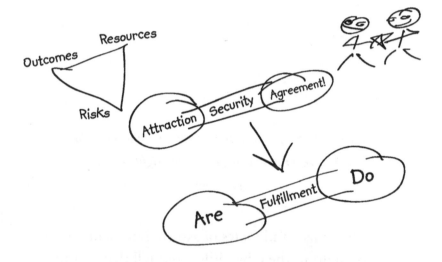

"We already agreed that for most adults, when work's good, life's better. Having a secure work role is a preliminary foundation, but it is not enough. You can see why first you must have or seek a work role that is, or will be, stable, dependable, reliable ..."

"… and that's accomplished by applying the Organizational Triangle to be competitively attractive to the organization combined with having clear agreement regarding all the factors of each corner," Cynthia interrupted.

"You got it! But, now we move to the other side of the work role equation, that is, your needs and requirements from work and career. RP begins to address this by separating who you 'are' from what you 'do.' Prying these two things apart is essential for us to discover 'fulfillment.' However, for many people this can be surprisingly difficult to accomplish. *Too many times, we lose our identity by incorrectly associating or confusing what we 'do' with who we 'are.' Those are two very different things!"* Elli was emphatic.

She continued, "What we elect to 'do' in our lives is, in part, made up of the many roles we play across time. We have work roles across our career. Equally, we have many other roles in other contexts of our lives such as friend, daughter, student, citizen, member, spouse, volunteer, mother and so forth. ***As to our work roles, what we 'do' is simply contextual personal performance and attention we are presently providing during a set time period or circumstance.*** Yes, 'Do' directly relates to the Organizational Triangle. But whatever this may be, it is only a tiny fraction of who we are, were and can be. When it comes to work, it's critical to fully discover who we 'are' so we can best consider our possibilities and choices as to what we can and should 'do.' Elli then began to draw another triangle next to the word **Are**, but this one was upside down compared to the Organizational Triangle.

"Let me guess, a personal framing for Work Role Mastery?" Cynthia was not at all hiding her anticipation to find out what this one was about. This might be what she had been looking for to guide her to the answers she had been seeking for many months.

"Correctamundo, my friend! This is the *Personal Triangle* ™ which is used to understand and map your life as it relates to your work. It is not intended to address all aspects of your life, just the parts of your being that pertain to, or are affected by, work and career. Anyone that works, or desires to work, has a Personal Triangle. Again, this is not what we 'do' but rather the much fuller and richer landscape of who we 'are.' This framework is a comprehensive way to explore the many facets of what you need from your work, as well as to evaluate the factors that should not be, or that you would prefer not to be, a part of your work. It is a way to uncover, recall and appraise all the values and qualities you might potentially offer to a work role's Organizational Triangle that you may not readily appreciate. The Personal Triangle is a way to create an inventory of possibilities and literally a wealth of knowledge enlightening us to our personal work-related factors and assets. The Personal Triangle begins to unveil the potential of predicting enjoyment, as well as dissatisfaction, at work."

Knowing they were running out of time this afternoon, Elli knew her pacing was important. She quickly
wrote words at each of the corners of the Personal Triangle:
I, We, and **Effects.**

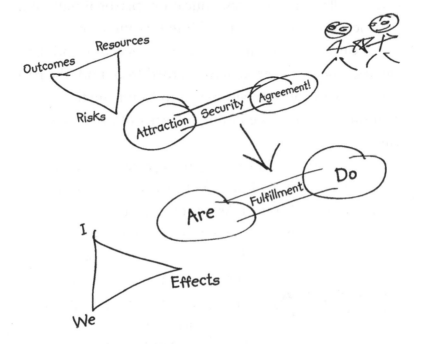

She then began, "Let me quickly run around the Personal Triangle with you. We'll begin with the 'I' corner.
**This is the corner containing all the factors that relate
directly or indirectly to work functions *in a personal
context.* This 'I' corner encompasses *everything that may
provide insights to your direct functional satisfaction or
dissatisfaction, as well as potentials of functional work
performance.*** These are the attributes and factors that

relate to functions you enjoy when doing them, as well as those you do not enjoy. This corner also includes an inventory and appraisal of the qualities you have to offer that an organization may functionally value and appreciate. This includes skills, competencies, education, personal traits and experiences related to functional interests and capabilities. We can learn much in this area through reflection and self-awareness, such as what we have learned from both the past and the present. We can also begin to formulate functional aspirations for our future in the 'I' corner of the Personal Triangle.

"This corner includes functional preferences and areas of curiosity. It includes functional aversions and activities you wish to avoid. It includes variety, or lack thereof, in your work functions. Just like in the Organizational Trian-

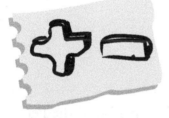

gle, understanding the negatives, or what we don't like, is just as important as understanding the positives, for we learn from both. This is also the corner that includes any functionally related personal strengths, weaknesses, values, ethics and especially the areas of our motivation. Other factors that matter are types of preferred functional thinking and problem-solving, the importance of repetition or lack of it, structure or lack of structure, physical activities, indoor and outdoor preferences and so forth that may relate to your 'I' corner. The scope and scale of accountability and responsibilities that one desires within their work role also resides in the 'I' area. Keep in mind, these may or may not be related directly to something that would be valued in a work role at the moment. However, all that you are, offer and know has the potential of raw and untapped elements of suitability or unsuitability for performing a function."

"So the 'I' corner is the heart of work enjoyment?"

"No, it's actually only a fraction of your needs regarding a satisfying work experience. This will make more sense as we look at the other two corners."

"OK, go on. I'm listening," said Cynthia.

The 'We' corner relates to the many social and interpersonal factors that may impact fulfillment and effectiveness in your work. This corner provokes you to think about all the people who surround and touch your work role in a direct manner. It makes you think about what they may mean to you and your life and career. This corner also encompasses a larger social perspective such as the organization's leadership, values, culture, industry, marketplace, mission and purpose. How you and other people interrelate is a really big deal and can have many positive and negative implications both in the moment as well as over the longer term. For example, consider how types, qualities, quantities, competencies, attitudes, enthusiasm and visions of people impact your happiness as well as your work performance. This corner reminds you to think about how the personalities, styles and characteristics of others are so relevant to you and how you view your work.

"But this corner is much more than just those concerns. One work role may bring you in contact with only the same people each day where you interact as a tightly woven team. On the other hand, another role may introduce to you total strangers in a wide variety of contexts and settings. Often work includes interactions with people outside of your organization. The social aspect of work is an important factor to personal performance and fulfillment, depending on your needs and capabilities. Think about how work can interplay with the diversity of co-workers, various styles of management, various types of customers, prospective customers, eager and aggressive suppliers or supporting professionals. For some, the *we* includes students, parents, criminals, patients, investors or even grieving families. Then there are the many social situations such as those with angry consumers, in combative situations or participating in challenging negotiations. Every work role has a range of social conditions and situations that should be taken into account by worker, supervisor and the designer of the work role."

Elli explained further, "For example, consider work role experiences serving happy customers all day who are savoring their new purchases, versus a workday of interaction with angry customers who are registering complaints due to product defects or delivery problems. Or think about the many types and forms of interpersonal elements of nurse, lawyer or police roles depending on their specific assignments and settings. Of course, the possible combinations are endless in this corner but considering their implications to you is paramount. There are no universal rights or wrongs per se, but the 'We' corner's design must be right for our desires, aversions, growth, comfort and stretch. Work roles should be chosen with the right social setting for unleashing our greatest potential and to ensure that we will be fulfilled simultaneously."

"So this corner is not what I do, but rather relates to all the people who are alongside me, as well as all those people that may influence or be influenced by my satisfaction and performance in my work? This includes all work interactions with people whether they are inside or outside of my organization, correct?" Cynthia questioned.

"Right on!" Elli answered. "This dimension of the Personal Triangle helps you to uncover the social conditions and situations that may be optimal for you, your career and your life. The 'We' corner may include the types of peers, clients, people in need of your help or care, vendors, advisors, professional groups, networks or communities that may be good, or not so good, for you. Perhaps more importantly for many of us, this corner may encompass the deeper purposes for our work if that work involves others, which it often does. This may be the reason for our passion at work, such as our ultimate sense of service to certain people, groups or mankind in general. Who we elect to serve may be inside or outside of our organizations. In any case, defining this as desirable and meaningful, or perhaps undesirable and meaningless, to us at this stage of our lives can be a vital part of self-discovery. This corner includes all aspects of the human ecosystem surrounding our work."

"This seems too big for me to even begin to think about!" Cynthia exclaimed.

"Once more, the Personal Triangle is simply a way of mapping *the reality you have* but may not appreciate. It helps you to better understand yourself so you can have a better and more enjoyable career. Let's slow down and just wade into the water, step by step."

"OK, sorry to be so dense," Cynthia apologized.

"Don't apologize. Each of the three Personal Triangle corners can seem overwhelming and strange at first, even though it is just a better way of appreciating ourselves, our needs and the 'whys of good work,'" Elli said in an encouraging manner and then returned to the topic. "In the most immediate and practical contexts, the 'We' corner includes the many personally relevant factors of person-to-person interactions and influences as you work each day. A work role typically places you within a team or department, among customers or suppliers, in organizations, industries, professions and marketplaces and many other categories of social interactivities and settings. On the other hand, some work roles may cause you to be isolated and quite independent from others. Of course, here I am describing generalities and extremes, but you get the point that all the social or 'We' factors are a really big deal as they concern our work.

"This corner is all about who you would like to have, or would like to avoid, as peers, who you desire to serve and be responsible to in your functional performance, as well as who might enjoy being accountable to perform for you. Certainly your direct manager or supervisor and their style of interaction and supervision can be an essential ingredient in both personal happiness and performance. This corner may include human interrelatedness upstream and downstream within processes, policies, regulations and procedures that may be a part of your work role. 'We' factors include things like whether you are asked to attend meetings and your role in those meetings and whether you will be asked to make presentations at those meetings. It includes management responsibilities, leading, coaching, enforcing, teaching, influencing, buying, negotiating or selling.

"Sometimes the work role's social environment characteristics, such as casual, formal, conflict, humor, seriousness, assertiveness, contention, danger, care-giving, helplessness, sophistication, trusting, mistrusting, tension, intensity or calmness, may influence your personal satisfaction or dissatisfaction in your work role."

The only ones among you who will be truly happy are
those who will have sought and found how to serve.
— Albert Schweitzer

Cynthia interjected, "Now I am starting to better understand what you are saying. In fact, I think the 'We' corner is one of the most important things that can bring me smiles or tears in my work. I can do almost anything when I am with the right group of people, but being with the wrong people makes me miserable. The people I work with, the purpose of our work and my work environment are three things that have kept me at my company in the last few years."

"So true! The people by our side as we fight the daily battles are so important. As you suggest, those we serve may be the reason for even fighting the battles. Equally, people can be primary or contributing reasons for frustration and despair in our work. It is up to each of us to know what is best for us socially in our work, then choose wisely and predictably," Elli affirmed, as a worker in the coffee shop dropped a cup. The sharp vibrations caused Elli to have an idea that might reinforce her points.

Elli instantly re-engaged. "Look at the workers moving about in this coffee shop at this moment. Think about how they might relate to each other, for better or worse. Look at their dependencies on each other, including the personal characteristics, even the impacts of moods that can lead to personal performance and enjoyment, as well as their collective productive synergy, or problematic liabilities. Observe their interplay together as they also constantly interact with customers of all types and demeanors; some are obviously regulars, while others seem to be strangers. Now think about how any given person might be really right, or might be really wrong for this work role setting. The activities we're observing in this coffee shop are a perfect example of what the 'We' corner is all about. Every organization is a tribe and you have to think a little like an anthropologist to fully appreciate that fact. Some people can find their way to becoming natives and others will always be misfits."

"Oh no, now Indiana Jones is a 'poster senior' for RP?" Cynthia laughed as she said this.

"Not exactly, but there's relevance, at least to the work of a real anthropologist. Interestingly, some of them are beginning to bring their science to organizations to help them figure this stuff out in a better way. The 'We' corner is about all those things related to human typologies, personalities and social situations that are your turn-ons and turn-offs. Just as no man is an island, work roles are not islands either. Or 'everybody's got to serve somebody,' as Bob Dylan said.

"Work roles are placed into a soup made up of other people, some within your organization and some outside of it. Depending on the setting, social factors can unleash your potential or extinguish it. This corner includes all the qualities and numbers of relationships you may have with associates, subordinates, trainees, examiners, inspectors, salespeople, buyers and so forth. For example, think of how many types of customer relationships there can be, ranging from consultative services that take place across decades like those of doctors, lawyers, dentists or accountants, versus just a few precious moments together on a phone in a call center. Additionally, all layers of leadership and management that are above and beside you reside in this corner, and particularly their philosophies, competencies, ethics, values and prac-

tices that may be suitable or unsuitable to you. Direct or matrixed reporting may have relevance to you and is in this corner. This corner includes community dynamics such as competitiveness, including direct one-to-one competition with co-workers, as well as team-to-team and industry competition."

"Wouldn't the two most important persons in the 'We' corner be your direct supervisor and the person leading the organization since those two can have such a positive or negative impact on you each day?" Cynthia asked, obviously pondering the topic.

"Frankly, I've never thought of it in that way, Cynthia, but that might be correct for many people and their circumstances," Elli answered. "Often your direct supervisor is the most critical single factor within the 'We' corner. This is why RP places so much emphasis on that person's competence in maintaining a good relationship with you. As to who you consider to be in second place to that person is a bigger question. For example, it might be your direct peers or maybe the nature, attitudes and qualities of your subordinates if you have management responsibilities. On the other hand, as you suggest, the CEO's vision and personal acumen may play a very significant part in setting the direction for your role and the working conditions, as well as your future with the organization.

"Related to this corner, keep in mind that the quality of communication and the communication venues and approaches used by the community is relevant, such as one-to-one conversational and spontaneous styles, e-mails versus group sessions, ways of collaboration and debate, open versus closed doors, noisy prairie dog cubicle cities versus privacy and the list goes on. How ideas and concerns are expressed can be paramount to some people's work morale, including both the ways of doing this and the timely, considerate responses to their expressions.

"Clearly this corner should include your diligent thinking about your personal preferences and aversions. Your thinking should also include assessing your potential strengths, assets, skills, education and experiences that may be highly valued by organizations regarding its social factors. In many roles, these can be some of the most valuable and appreciated qualities you bring to them. But, as in all parts of the Personal Triangle, remember there's no general or universal right answers for everyone here, but rather each person must decide what is best for them."

"I'm with you on that," Cynthia agreed, then added, "different strokes for different folks ..."

"Ain't that the truth?" Elli expressed, pounding her fist on the table with a humorous, exaggerated twang. Then she continued, "All three Personal Triangle corners hold clues and information that are predictive of personal success or failure, as well as happiness or despair. *Self-knowledge is critical and must be applied for well-informed and diligent decision-making as you choose work roles and their environments. The inherent nature and characteristics of interactions between you and the other persons you interact with each day will have a tremendous impact on your personal satisfaction or dissatisfaction at work.* Of course, in most roles, the competence or incompetence of others will impact you in many ways!"

"That I painfully know!" Cynthia validated.

"Me too! Workplace enthusiasm and esprit de corps can be really important to some of us. Humor and laughter may be a turn-on or a turn-off as we work. Some folks enjoy a highly competitive community, while others like to be in highly cooperative and collaborative circumstances. Some are loners needing freedom and independence. At the other extreme, others prefer to be social butterflies, engaged in closely-knit networks with fellow workers, patients, students, customers or vendors. Some like to have authority and responsibility over others, some do not. Some can flourish being immersed in danger, death and disease, others cannot. Some work best on a team at the same place and in the same way each day, others do best as roaming mavericks on the road. And then others perform optimally with the flexibility of working remotely at home while still being an integral part of a team. Most of us reside somewhere between these extremes on continuums; there are endless situational variables."

> *To different minds, the same world is a hell and a heaven.*
> — Ralph Waldo Emerson

Elli continued, "Some workers relish highly diverse social settings that are a melting pot of human differences, while others like to be in more homogeneous teams where everyone thinks and behaves in a similar manner. The actual size or the age of an organization can be important to many, since there are many experiential differences between a small, entrepreneurial new venture and a large, multinational organization. Relatedly, there are many differences between the generational family-run organizations and publicly-held corporations."

Elli began to wrap up this topic, "At the most basic level, the 'We' corner relates to where your work role 'resides' within the bigger picture. You can think of this corner as the 'village' surrounding the work functions of your 'I' corner." Elli was highly animated as she made consecutive quote marks with her hands when she emphasized, *resides*, *I* and *village*. She continued, "By the very nature of a work role, you are plugging yourself into a work community, a culture and an industry. As you do so, it's gotta be a good fit for you and you gotta be a good fit for the village."

"It seems to me that 'We' is the most important corner, even more important than what I do in my tasks and functions," Cynthia said with the confidence of a novice.

"Maybe, maybe not. That's for you to decide since any such conclusion would be totally subjective. But before you rush to judgment, there's still another corner to cover. You might find it to be even more important. Personally I think all three corners hold equal importance and offer vast, unexplored potential to most workers, although we seldom seek to discover this diligently and rigorously." Elli cautioned, "People and work roles each have their own respective characteristics. What's so sad and dangerous is that there is often so little thought given to these important factors by workers, candidates, recruiters or management. People and their work roles should be well matched, much better than is generally done today. This is the responsibility of both parties. But yes, you are right that the 'We' corner is very important to most of us. Finding good social fit in our work roles is a must for most of us to be truly happy in our work. I'm also hopeful that you better appreciate now how all the other people within this corner have direct impact on our work performance, thus our career security. Again, don't forget to look at *both sides* of this corner to discover your positives and negatives. It's as important to understand what we do not want as it is to know what we do want in our interpersonal interactions and work environments. Everything can be very good in both the 'I' or 'We' corners, but you can still be miserable at work due to problems or conflicts in the other corner, or perhaps in the corner yet to come."

"Wow, so true!" Cynthia exclaimed. "Both have to be right, don't they? I really like the 'We' of my work for the most part. It's the 'I' that seems to be such a mess for me lately. This is so much clearer now."

"RP principles do open your eyes. These two Triangle frameworks are strong diagnostic tools which help you to achieve self-discovery, solve problems, find remedies and make opportunities more visible. It is up to you to understand who you are, what you need and the values you can offer to a work role's Organizational Triangle so that it's right for you based on the inventory and qualities you have in your Personal Triangle. As you can see, you are already starting to use the common language of RP. Just imagine if you could talk about this stuff at work everyday and if everyone were familiar with the language and the principles."

"That's almost unimaginable!"

"Actually, it's quite possible and practical. All you have to do is add a little literacy in your life and workplace about the realities of work. But remember, there's still one more corner, 'Effects.' This corner is just as important as the first two corners for most workers and candidates. As the name somewhat implies, *this corner addresses all the factors in the other parts of one's life that are impacted by our work role. In the other direction, it also encompasses the other parts of our life that may need to impact or have influence upon our work.* These are the acceptable and unacceptable or desirable and undesirable factors that go from our work outward into our life or those that come from our life into our work."

Elli added, "For example, this includes the quality of life and standard of living our role provides to us and our family. It also includes the influences that are allowed on our work such as children and flex time for parenting or perhaps eldercare. This area encompasses all that we want to derive in all aspects of our life that are related to, or are caused by, our work. Here you find issues, if they exist, regarding shifts, part-time, overtime, weekend work and travel. This is where compensation and benefits often reside, though sometimes these may fit in other corners for some people as well. There may be factors in this corner that make you more attractive, such as being able to travel, being able to work weekends or overtime, desiring professional development and career advancement, having extensive personal networks that may benefit the organization, and so forth."

Elli continued, "Tuition assistance for you or your children or being able to leave work occasionally for a school play or a sick child, reside in this corner. Healthcare, fitness and other forms of assistance programs are in the 'Effects' corner. This corner also includes the related support and respect you have, or don't have, for a work role or profession from your spouse, significant others, friends or even the community-at-large. Even the media can have significant impact on our image of our work. Just ask teachers, soldiers or police. Conditions such as relocation requirements, geographic location and all that may be included within a geographic area are in this corner. Commute time, hassles and costs are here, as well as parking ease or difficulty. Pertinent personal income and property taxes are in this corner as well as the underlying financial stability of the work role or the organization across time.

"The 'Effects' corner brings to our attention how imperative it is that a work role must fit well into our chosen and best-lived life, not the other way around. Equally, this corner also brings to our attention how our lives sometimes will need to flex, adapt and respond to the realities of the chosen work roles that we determine to place into our lives. That's especially true when we select less desirable roles in the short term as a stepping stone to another more desirable role in the longer term. We may make compromises for a period of time or for other reasons and situations that exist in our life. This can be an area that amplifies our satisfaction or even the deeper reasons for our work for some of us. This can be a corner that correlates with severe underlying tensions and causes anxiety regarding our work roles. For example, heavy debt, spouse relocation, needing to be in the proximity of relatives or other significant obligations in our life can sometimes force us to make tough choices. All of these are a part of the 'Effects' corner. As in all corners of both Triangles, exploring the negatives, or what we don't want to occur, is just as important as exploring the positives, or what we do desire. We must look at both sides in order to gain complete understanding."

Cynthia now was astounded. "I have simply never thought of each of these areas of me, or me at work, and their interplay related to both happiness and the rest of my life. Again, it's obvious in retrospect, especially looking at all of this simultaneously. I now see that it's not enough to address just one of these corners. To be satisfied, you must consider all of them. It's like a heavy fog is lifting!"

"Very good. Remember, there are no rights or wrongs in this corner except that which is right or wrong for you. It's your Personal Triangle. It's important that you know each corner well so that you are aware of the best ways to market yourself as well as your work role decisions. Each corner of the Personal Triangle should be a good fit with each corner of the Organizational Triangle. *It's generally not realistic to have every corner of the Personal Triangle perfect all the time, but you do have to diligently try to construct your work roles so that you are making correct, well-informed compromises.*

"The factors within your Personal Triangle are also relative in their importance to you at this point in your life. Across your life, your Personal Triangle is often changing. In each corner, there will be *core* factors that may be variable and flexible depending on the situation. There will be some things that are in your *inventory* that you do not wish to ap-

ply presently but can call upon if you should need, such as a skill, experience or knowledge. And then there will be *Screamers*. Screamers are those factors or conditions that are absolutely imperative to you and thus are non-negotiable. In any case, it is critical we understand that we each have needs, requirements, qualities, values, attributes, preferences, aversions and pertinent situations in all three of these corners. The Personal Triangle can provide us with self-discoveries and insights about ourselves that will assist with our decisions relating to work and career."

"Cynthia, in the interest of time, I'm afraid I have oversimplified all of this, so you need to read *Career Fulcrum* as soon as I can get it to you."

"I understand," Cynthia assured.

"Keep in mind, the Personal Triangle, just like the Organizational Triangle, does not provide the answers. Each are more like treasure maps which can be used to help you learn more about yourself and your work role situation, to ask the right questions and to look in the right places for answers. *The Organizational Triangle will lead to understanding the organizational domains of work. The Personal Triangle will lead to understanding your personal domains regarding work. They are both value-neutral. There are no rights or wrongs, per se. That is for you and your organization to decide and choose. The Triangles are excellent ways to better organize thoughts related to work, career and the personal marketing of your qualities to gain what you seek.*"

"Now I can see how all you've shared would allow anyone to diagnose their work roles and improve their careers with accuracy and effectiveness. I'm also now starting to see how you can actually form an agreement. *It would be very hard to create a workable agreement without this structure and the construct of a work role, wouldn't it?*" Cynthia questioned, almost rhetorically.

Elli responded, "Yes, very hard, but we're not finished yet. RP educates and enables us to better respond to our realities related to our work. Because of this, RP can also serve as an important diagnostic tool when we are searching for remedies and solutions for making things work better for you and the organization. Keep in mind, there's still more to come. Right now, we are only talking about the 'Are' side of Fulfillment. Let's quickly go over and take a peek at the 'Do' side before our husbands send out a search party for us."

Elli resumed, "Every Personal Triangle is as unique and complex as the person it represents. Once you do the deep digging and exploration that is required for better understanding, you will want to think next about the 'Do' side of the Fulfillment equation." She then pointed to the word on the other side of Fulfillment.

The problem is not that there are problems. The problem is expecting otherwise and thinking that having problems is a problem.
— Theodore Rubin

TEN

DESIGNING WORK FULFILLMENT

If I had eight hours to chop down a tree, I'd spend six
sharpening my ax.
— Abraham Lincoln

E lli now explained the two sides of 'Do,' which to
many could be complex and confusing at first.
"The Organizational Triangle represents 'Do,' *but*
only from the organizational viewpoint. Attention to the
organization's viewpoint provides you with security, as we
talked about before, with attraction and agreement. 'Do'
must also be considered from your viewpoint, for by doing
so, you can gain greater fulfillment in your work. Fulfillment demands that you match all the functions and circumstances of your work role as closely as possible to the traits,

desires, aversions, assets, factors and qualities within each of the three corners of your Personal Triangle. Assuring that your Personal Triangle is well fitted to your work role will generate satisfaction across your career. There are many approaches and methods to accomplishing this objective. Being diligent in understanding and documenting each Personal Triangle corner is an excellent beginning.

"Of course, this also entails determining just how much of your life you desire to allocate to your work, not just in time, but in purpose, energy and attention, which, by the way, would technically be in the Personal Triangle's 'Effects' corner. *Career Fulcrum* provides a *Work Role Experience Assessment*™ that allows you to accurately predict the

degree of satisfaction you will have performing each aspect of a specific work role."

"You can accurately predict enjoyment in your work? Like, in advance?" Cynthia was fascinated with that prospect.

"Absolutely, if you know your Personal Triangle and if you're well informed about the work role beforehand. *Career Fulcrum* also offers something called the *Eight Dimensions*™ that provides a variety of ways to adjust work roles to better suit a Personal Triangle, as well as to fit better with an Organizational Triangle. But for now, there are a couple of quick ways to help you begin to think about matching your Personal Triangle needs to what you 'do' at work. You should always try to design your work for maximum enjoyment. Fulfilling work is not usually achieved by luck, fate or accident."

"Design my work?"

"Sure. You, your work and the organization are too important to approach it in any other way. Enjoyment in your work is not selfishness either, since that's the way you will always perform the best. When you are happier in your work, you will be successful and the organization will be better rewarded. There are plenty of roles, conditions and situations out there so everyone can ultimately find work role relationships that please them. When a worker or candidate and the organization have ample understanding to make wise selection decisions about each other, they can predictably form durable, highly productive, satisfying relationships. Let me show you a little about 'Flow' and I think you'll see possibilities for work design much better." Again Elli quickly drew a simple diagram below Fulfillment. It had two arrows, one on the x axis going left to right and one on the y axis going bottom to top, again labeled 'Are' and 'Do,' with a Zone called **Flow** at a 45 degree angle, and on either side, an **A Zone** and a **B Zone.**

"Flow?" Cynthia's questions kept coming.

Adding more to her graphic, Elli returned to her student's urgently needed instruction. She was just about out of time. "Whenever your 'are,' or you might say the completeness of your Personal Triangle, is well-balanced with your 'do,' you can achieve a state of Flow. Keep in mind, that in this case, 'Do' is the entirety of the work role, including its functions that take place in environments and situations. This concept of Flow was originated by professor Mihaly Csikszentmihalyi at the University of Chicago. He has extensively researched what leads people to 'optimal experiences' in their lives. Flow is the term he coined for these optimal experiences. I urge you to read his book, *Finding Flow*. Good work should provide us with Flow, at least most of the time. When you are experiencing Flow you're deeply satisfied."

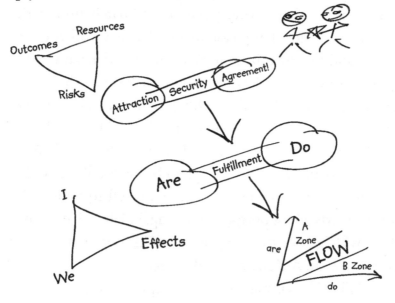

Elli added, "Typically, there is the right amount of stress, challenge, stimulation or stretch, and you are performing at peak levels. *While in Flow, you are more curious, enthusiastic, engaged, alert in the function and deeply inter-*

ested in what you are doing. The functions you are performing have your total attention. You tend to lose your sense of self, place and time. You are lost in your work, or you could say you are 'one with your work.' You find yourself being more creative and far more productive when you are in Flow. It's a very good place. You are happier. Some athletes, actors and musicians refer to this as being in 'The Zone.'"

"I've been there many times. I know the feeling and you're right, it's a very good place to be. But having those kinds of experiences on a regular basis is something that hasn't happened for a long time," Cynthia recalled. "In fact, that's what's been missing in my work!"

"Knowing what's missing is a good start. Now we need to figure out what's wrong or what's the cause." Elli had been taught never rush to conclusions, no matter how tempting. "RP teaches to always *seek understanding first, and to do so by applying ample humility. As they say, 'enjoy your ignorance!'* Let's talk about 'Are' and 'Do' using this x/y diagram. Simply stated, 'Are' is your Personal Triangle in its entirety and 'Do' is your work role. *Whenever the relative make-up of your Personal Triangle, or your 'are,' exceeds what you are being asked to 'do' in your role, this places you into the A Zone.* This may be when your work role is not challenging or stretching you enough. You 'are' more than your work. You could say your capacities, motivations and interests exceed your assignments and responsibilities. *The A Zone is a place of boredom, disengagement and restlessness.* It's not a good place to be for long.

"On the other hand, *when what you are being asked to 'do' exceeds your 'are,' which again is your present and relative Personal Triangle makeup, you find yourself in the B Zone. The symptoms of the B Zone can be excessive or toxic stress, despair, low self-esteem, overwhelmed, loss of confidence and high levels of anxiety.* Your work role's demands are exceeding who you 'are' or your capabilities and qualities, at least at the moment.

"Notice both dimensions of the diagram are represented with arrows. This is to indicate the changing nature of people and work roles. For most of us, our 'are,' that is our Personal Triangle, is seldom static. You are growing, developing, learning, experiencing, maturing and moving through different chapters and stages of life. Likewise, on the 'do' side, some work roles are seldom static and are typically filled with all forms of changes. Some are more static than others. *As you can readily imagine, the rate of change of the person versus the rate of change of the role can generate a constant enjoyment. Conversely, these dynamics can create a variety of problematic situations when there are significant mismatches between the two dimensions.*

"In any case, it is normal that one will normally drift in and out of Flow with time, even during a day as different functions are performed. *The key is trying to stay in the Flow Zone as much as reasonable.* For example, it is typical that upon entering a new role or a new work environment, you may be within the B Zone for a while, until your 'Are' catches up with your 'Do,' so to speak. On the other hand, if your role does not change, or if you grow faster than your role, such as your capabilities, motivations and interests, etc., you may drop out into the A Zone. It is typical that you may have momentary excursions into the A Zone and the B Zone in most work roles, but the majority of time should be in Flow. It is possible some people have never experienced Flow in their work. *It is also critical that your Flow Zone accurately and consistently overlays the functions that the organization seeks to be performed well. If not, Flow can place you in major jeopardy, since you will be enjoying doing what the organization does not desire for you to be doing.*"

"Eureka, Elli! I'm in the A Zone! I'm not in Flow. And I've been in the A Zone for quite some time and didn't even know it. Elli, you are a miracle worker!" Cynthia proclaimed.

"Hey girl, I'm just the messenger. This simple RP diagnostic tool deserves the credit. But remember, you still may not know why you are in the A Zone and out of Flow. *These three Zones are only symptoms or effects of underlying causes.* You need to know what is putting you into the A Zone, and you also need to understand what may place you into Flow. You're going to have to look deep into your Personal Triangle to find out why your present role is boring you as well as what your needs are. Then as you do so, perhaps you can adjust or modify your work role, by agreement, to get you back into Flow. You already have a big clue though. If you are in the A Zone, it is because you are more than the present role you are doing. You may need more challenge. But to find what that might be, you've got to explore your own Personal Triangle. Based on what you are saying, I suggest you look for discoveries in the 'I' and 'We' corners of your Personal Triangle. Can you now appreciate how all these frameworks are used together as a whole set of tools to allow you to have Work Role Mastery?"

"Yes, I can clearly see that. I'm really getting a tremendous amount from your guidance today, Elli," Cynthia said, expressing gratitude.

"Thanks, but again, it's just RP being applied to your life. Now we are finally on the home stretch. There's just one more thing I want to bring to your attention because it may be helpful tonight as you think about all of this. In addition to *Career Fulcrum*, which is the basic handbook and manual for a worker or candidate to practice RP, there is another book I advise as a fine complement. It's *Happier* by Tal Ben-Shahar. You may have heard of it already because it's also the text for the most popular course at Harvard University. And why not, life's all about being happier, right?"

"Right," Cynthia said smiling. By this point she had written an amazing number of notes for such a brief period of time.

Elli was now drawing again, placing three overlapping circles next to 'Do.' "Whatever you elect to do as a work role, you should always consider three interrelated components of being happier in your work. Each of these again can be determined by understanding your Personal Triangle.

Briefly these are: *What work, or 'Do,' will give you life meaning? What work, or 'Do,' will provide you with pleasure? What work, or 'Do,' will make the best use of your personal strengths?"*

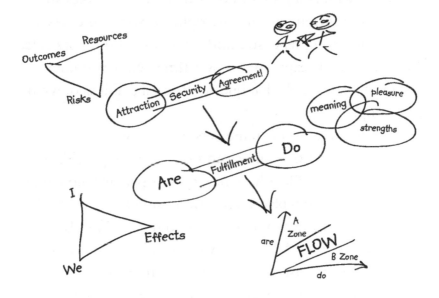

"This is known as the **MPS model ... meaning, pleasure** and **strengths.** MPS provides a greater depth to the 'Do' side to ensure that you will have the keys to fulfillment."

Elli continued, *"Happier* provides much more about the merit and method of MPS. This book will also provide valuable insights and general guidance for becoming happier. But, as it relates to work, and as you already anticipate I'm sure, all of these answers are to be found within the three corners of your Personal Triangle. Don't forget, it's essential that you rigorously explore both the positive and negative aspects of each corner, for only then will you gain a more complete understanding. Then you couple self-awareness with being well-informed about work roles and forming the agreements that are right for you. Of course, this requires comprehensive understanding of the work role, its nature and its expectations over time. Now you know what to look for and what questions to ask," Elli said, wrapping it up.

"Elli, I am not the same person that I was a couple of hours ago when I first came into this coffee shop. This is all incredible! It's like I have new eyes or perhaps more like I have had a brain replacement. Every single part of Work Role Mastery is essential knowledge to survive in today's workplace, isn't it? And those two Triangles are dynamite guidance for the basic aspects of a work role relationship."

"Now you can see why I've been so bullheaded about telling you about RP, Cynthia! As I've said, RP explains work's realities. You're now seeing work in a more complete and accurate way." Elli felt a sense of relief. She was confident that Cynthia was going to be fine.

"I've believed in RP's power because it describes and applies reality, instead of promoting hollow motivational dogma or 'rah-rah' fads," Elli said. "It remodels our points of view, and in fact, it remodels work. *It does not provide the answers, for that is our responsibility. But it does provide principle-based structure and precipitates the right questions.* It's also the only approach I've experienced equally serving and assisting both the worker's and the organization's interest in a neutral, effective manner. That is so important because both are equally incentivized to be responsive to the other. *Work's a we thing!*"

"As it should," Cynthia chimed in.

Suddenly, Elli offered a caution in a rather strong tone that caught Cynthia a little off guard. *"Keep in mind, Relationship Performance gives you excellent theory and powerful tools, but it is your responsibility to apply it effectively.* Just like in carpentry, engineering or medicine, great theory and dependable tools are the right beginnings, but they do not in themselves provide you with the *realization* of what you desire. You must utilize them with the right thought, judgment and actions. For example, latent power, as well as security, is achieved by applying the Organizational Triangle as a fulcrum for leverage throughout your career. But don't depend upon that principle alone to make good things happen for you. *To enjoy the power of the Organizational Triangle, you have to stand tall and effectively articulate what you want. Don't expect anyone to know what you need or to be responsive to your needs unaided or undirected or without effective nudges in the right direction. You must express your needs authentically and effectively."*

After saying this, Elli finished her drawing by adding another bar with a circle on either end. She labeled the line

Realization, and then wrote **Choice** and **Predictability** in the circles in the same manner as she had before with Security and Fulfillment.

Elli explained, "As you apply the Organizational Triangle within Agreement, you will be inevitably valued, respected, and reasonably secure, barring unforeseen circumstances. However, just because you are secure or valued does not mean the organization will be necessarily forthcoming or responsive in satisfying your own needs. Indeed, how can they even be aware of them?"

Elli continued, "This is an important point that relates directly to getting what you need, and by this I mean *within the constraints of reason and merit.*"

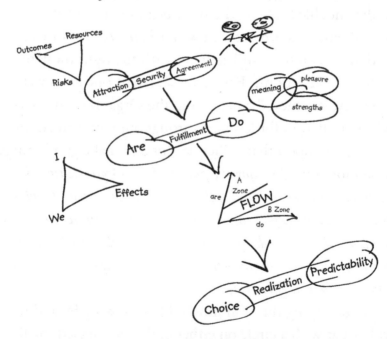

Elli went on, "Realize means to 'make real' or to 'make reality.' To realize your requirements from work, you must effectively express your needs to gain organizational responsiveness to them. Simply possessing greater, but passive, self-awareness of your needs, such as those new discoveries by using Personal Triangle mapping or those that are gained by applying Flow and MPS diagnostics are not enough to make your needs realized. And effective expression goes far beyond simply articulating your needs. *Effectiveness in gaining what you reasonably desire requires a willingness to exercise the power of choice and predictability you possess in order to gain the organization's attention and responsiveness.*

"Each party's natural momentum is to care foremost for their own needs. Organizations are distracted away from your needs because they are focused upon their needs. You will not gain their attention and responsiveness unless you present your compelling argument from a position of strength. If you are accepting and tolerant of inattention and unresponsiveness to your reasonable needs, expect nothing else. You are back to depending on luck and fate again. How could you expect otherwise? Why would anyone give anything else if they get what they need without giving anything else?"

"They wouldn't. I've seen that happen so many times. I'm even guilty of it myself," Cynthia affirmed.

Elli was now wrapping up her instruction. "So the third area of Work Role Mastery is *realization*. To realize what you seek in a work role, you must apply both *choice* and *predictability*. It's an abundant world today that's filled with attractive options for high-performance talent, just as organizations have plenty of options as well. Your constant goal should be ensuring that you and your organization have the realization of a healthy and rewarding work role relationship with each other. This will only happen if you speak up and share your needs and desires honestly, completely and authentically with the organization and vice versa. You will only tend to do this consistently and forthrightly if you appreciate that you have choices and can exercise them with predictability."

> *Our lives begin to end the day we remain silent about*
> *things that matter.*
> — Martin Luther King Jr.

"*Of course this always needs to be done upon a secure foundation of attractive, agreed upon work role performance, or the promise thereof, in each corner of the work role's Organizational Triangle.* Do not expect the organization to read your mind, nor provide for your needs because of altruism and good will. But here's the secret to this—you will never be an effective advocate for your own needs unless you constantly understand and consider your options. If you believe you have no other options, you will find yourself in the cruel, tortured world of a 'scarcity mindset.' Sure, it's an artificial world, but seems as if it is real for many people. Scarcity mindset occurs when someone is not willing to create, entertain and consider their other options. They either fail to be a top performer in the way the Organizational Triangle demands and/or they keep their mouth shut and accept whatever comes their way ... whether modest, mediocre or downright ugly."

Elli's instruction continued, *"This does not, by any means, imply that you should be unreasonable in your requests and requirements, inappropriately demanding or irrational in what you seek. Nor does it mean that you should not apply good judgment with due compromise, patience and flexibility.* However, it does mean that being responsive to the Organizational Triangle leads to power and options in an abundant talent marketplace. These provide you with choice. In this marketplace, both parties must be competitively attractive, and by being so, they apply their attractiveness to get what they seek, within the realm of reason. *Competition benefits both parties, though this may be hard to accept initially. It can be hard to appreciate that you actually do the organization a disservice by not expressing your needs."*

Elli went on, "Only by articulating your needs will they become better in being attractive to you, thus getting the best performance from you and  having more durable relations with you. It works much like the retail marketplace—competition makes for better products at better value. In the workplace, competition makes for better work role relationships, performance, innovation and personal satisfaction. Too many workers and organizations have been far too complacent, indifferent and lethargic toward each other for far too long. They have operated as if they or the other party does not have alternative options. They have failed to exercise their power of choice to make things better. It has often caused harm to both. *Reciprocal choice facilitates reciprocal performance."*

Cynthia interjected, "That's a hard edge, isn't it?"

Elli countered, "Not really. It's neither hard nor soft, but just a better theory about today's reality. Both parties have choices and both must rise correctly and effectively to the occasion. Compassion and good will for each other should exist. There should be no maliciousness or ill intent. Nothing about RP is zero sum. You have abundant choices you can exercise inside your organization and beyond its walls, and so does the organization. Neither party will reliably gain what they seek unless they pursue work role relationship agreements with other optional choices as their backdrop.

"This means agreements must be derived from straight-talk and a shared philosophy that *work's a we thing.* Both parties must be willing to pursue their other best options if they cannot obtain reasonable responsiveness and flexibility from the other party. This makes each better and more attentive to the other. Doing work this way gets everything into the open so that there's no festering or surprises for anyone. *Simple straight talk can cure many illnesses in the workplace.* This way both parties accurately serve the other because it is clearly in their best self-interest to do so. It's somewhat like a new form of Adam Smith's two hundred year old 'Invisible Hand,' but for the workplace. Work is a free market. In choice there is power. To achieve realization, you must have more than only one option, for only then is there choice, which you see in my drawing."

Cynthia looked down and said, "And predictability?"

"Yes," Elli confirmed, "Choice is useless, squandered or ineffective if you cannot apply predictability for making good decisions. Without predictability, choice is simply like gambling at the roulette wheel. That can lead to reluctance and inhibitions as to doing the right thing. *Having good judgment about what will be good or bad for you within work role agreements, or reaching good decisions comparing different work roles, is impossible without applying predictability.* Look again at the entirety of this Work Role Mastery framing. Carefully reconsider the predictive power of the Organizational Triangle, the Personal Triangle, Agreement, Flow and MPS. Consider how all of these can be brought together in synthesis to provide you with both predictable security and fulfillment. Can you see that these principles not only allow you to understand the whole landscape of work better, but now you have all the ingredients to make better decisions based upon being more self-aware and informed?"

"Yes, without any doubt or gambling as you aptly put it," Cynthia responded.

Elli continued, "Gaining ample information for accurate understanding through the use of reliable principles is vital for predictability. *To summarize, to have the **realization** of **security** and **fulfillment**, you must apply **choice** and **predictability**. This may seem a little abstract, the way we are hurrying through this, but I think you'll soon see what I mean. Indeed, how can you even collaborate on and reliably enter into a work role agreement with an organization without security and fulfillment being more predictable? Applying choice and predictability in this manner will make it much more probable that you realize a durable, rewarding work role relationship."*

"This is really interesting. I can see how this can be so true," Cynthia reflected. "It's like the forces of choice cause both parties to do the right things for the other, which in turn creates the right rewards for them. It's up to me to be a great value to the organization, but I am accountable to also clearly and fully express my needs. But if I do not see that I have choices that I can pursue with predictability, I am not empowered. Rather, I am just drawing cards. Therefore, I will not be able to form a reasonable agreement that serves both parties' best interests. I can also envision this will require a higher quality of communication between the worker and their Talent Steward, or straight talk, as I think you say."

"You got it!" Elli exclaimed. "*It benefits no one if you exit an organization because they were unresponsive to your needs. However, it's your responsibility to express them and to balance your needs well against their Organizational Triangle needs. It is wasteful or sad whenever anyone is terminated because the organization or the worker failed to effectively un-*

leash their full potential together within a work role. It just makes sense that you must express your needs thoughtfully, considerately and in a spirit of good will and by forming agreement. Often, this takes a combination of *personal assertiveness* and *reasoned temperance.* Yes, I realize those can be opposites. Typically, this just means you have to stand tall and be of great value. Then articulate your needs and negotiate with reasonable patience, empathy, creativity and flexibility. It is a balancing act, but using RP's dependable principles and practical common sense within quality dialog is always the best approach." Elli was feeling a sense of accomplishment in her impromptu instruction.

> *The most important distinction between aggression and assertion is its intent. During assertion, we move ourselves toward another; during aggression, we move ourselves against another. Assertion is vital within a relationship.*
> — Georgia Lanoil

Cynthia again asked to review her understanding. Elli invited her to do so. Again, she demonstrated that she had been a perfect student. She nailed every aspect, point and part of the entire Work Role Mastery set of frameworks. In fact, she was rather amazing. Clearly she had a lot to offer to organizations. As she closed her book of notes, Cynthia said, "I have so much to think about this evening that my head might burst. I'm skipping the gym tonight!"

Elli replied, "Just take it step by step, my friend. It's all going to get back on track now. RP will take you to the place you want to go."

"I think you're right, Elli. Again, thank you so much for all that you've shared this afternoon. I owe you big time."

"My day will come and I won't be bashful. You know that." Elli smiled, confident that whatever that day she referred to was about, it was unlikely to be about work. But then she reflected—life holds so many other dimensions beyond work, each chock full of surprises waiting to be revealed.

They began putting everything away. As they were leaving the table, heading to the door and out to their cars, Cynthia inquired, "I believe I can apply these frameworks to begin moving toward a work role relationship with Rick tomorrow. I'm sold on RP. Now I need to get it into our organization. How do we begin to put RP into practice?"

If you deliberately set out to be less than you are
capable, you'll be unhappy for the rest of your life.
— Abraham Maslow

ELEVEN

OUTFITTING

What is the hardest task in the world? To think.
— Ralph Waldo Emerson

Walking out to their cars, they silently savored a beautiful sunset. Distant winds were using the sun's receding light to paint varying hues upon high, wispy clouds. Venus was just becoming visible in a section of darker sky. This was a perfect backdrop for such an important afternoon, Cynthia thought.

"What a day! So you're going to get me a copy of *Career Fulcrum*, right?" Cynthia nudged.

"Yep, in fact, you can even get it tonight at the website, www.rpPaQ.com. Also at the web site, you'll learn about *QR*™," Elli said, distracted, unlocking her car.

"QR? Something else to learn?" Cynthia responded with a faked outburst, only half-jokingly, her head down and arms outstretched for effect.

"Not really. QR simply means *quality of relationship*. QR's a fast way for you and Rick to understand the powerful, bi-directional forces of work quality. QR combines the Personal Triangle and the Organizational Triangle into a single, six-sided *structure to describe and measure the core elements of a work relationship. You've always had QR in place with Rick, for better or worse. You and Rick just didn't know it or have a way to measure it.* I suspect that you've each based work too much upon assumptions and misinformation, and that's way too dangerous for any worker, supervisor or leader in today's workplace.

"I bet much of what you and Rick need to get on better footing with each other is this QR framework. By using this method, each of you will have the important factors of your work relationship better illuminated in monthly QR Snapshots. It's a reliable, easy way for you to express and know where you stand with each other, and to do so accurately and fast.

"By having a measurable structure of work quality, what were once difficult conversations will now become much easier. QR brings attention to those parts of your relationship that require dialog, while desensitizing the messy emotional stuff, or the non-relevant things, that can trip you up. In just a few minutes at the beginning of each month, you share perspectives with each other online. You and Rick become far more alert and tuned-in to each other's realities. When needed, you seek remedies for anything that's not optimal for either of you."

Cynthia quizzed, "So you're saying QR summarizes all we've talked about tonight into one simple online picture? Now you tell me this?" Cynthia placed ample emphasis on "this?"

"Well, I wouldn't go so far as to say everything we've discussed. But it's true that periodic QR Snapshots are a giant leap forward for creating *better work in better lives*™. You should think of a QR Snapshot as the vital signs of work wellness and career security, much as blood pressure and temperature are vital signs for your health. And just like medical vital signs, QR Snapshots are not the deeper diagnostics. You seek those discoveries by having dialog whenever your QR Snapshot alerts you that there's a need to do so."

"Elli, I believe we really can—no, I believe we *must* do this, not just for Rick and me, but for the good of our company and everyone who works here!" Cynthia was visibly excited.

"Now you can see why I'm such an evangelist! Just can't help myself," Elli said laughing. "Maybe I made this too difficult tonight. Tell Rick I'll be glad to help him get RP underway. It's best to have small, open discussions upfront, like you and I did this evening, so viewpoints, doubts and ideas can be shared between workers and supervisors.

He can find a discussion guide and other tips at the web site.

"Everyone has three online rpPaQ tools. One, called *rpCamera*™, captures and reveals QR information each month in a *QR Snapshot*™. Another, *rpMat*™, is a checklist for having better diagnostic and remedy-seeking dialogs with each other whenever needed. And *rpWeaver*™ is the third tool. Like we've discussed, rpWeaver creates work relationship agreements in a balanced, collaborative online process. Everyone uses the same tools and, get this—everyone is offered the same guidance and support, whether they're worker, supervisor or leader. Is that radical or what?" Elli exclaimed.

"Those tools, plus treating everyone in a workplace equally, sound very different, and very cool!"

"They are! In RP everyone is outfitted to have the "we thing" at work. But remember, your leadership must be committed to the principles of Relationship Performance. This means leadership accepting, supporting and promoting *shared accountability* for creating and maintaining *better work in better lives*. No one's entitled or exempt from accountability any longer. But there's nothing about RP that's hard ... *if* folks want things to truly improve at work and in life. It only requires a sincere desire to get better, a shift in thinking that's grounded in reality and a willingness from both parties to become more attentive and attractive to each other's reasonable needs. Oh yes, one more thing, each must remember they always possess *the power of choice* as to what they will, and will not, accept."

"Knowing that you have choice is crucial, isn't it?" Cynthia said in a low voice, as if speaking only to herself.

"Yep, choice is the cornerstone of shared accountability. *Choice is the underlying force that propels stronger work relationships.* The tools enable you to be better informed, a better thinker, performer and communicator, plus you are more secure in your work role. With these you more accurately do what's best so that you have greater power in choosing your work's rewards.

"Consider how your thinking has changed tonight. Imagine what would happen if every supervisor, leader and worker at your company only knew what you know at this moment, then were each equipped with tools to make work better and to prevent dangerous assumptions. RP's so rewarding and prudent for everyone to practice. And in case you're wondering, RP doesn't consume more of anyone's precious time. In fact, RP actually provides more time, since everyone spends less of their time 'fighting fires,' doing the wrong things or compensating for chronic dysfunctions. RP's the best investment your organization may ever make."

"Maybe the second best," Cynthia teased, displaying a newfound perspective. "I'm going to be the best investment they'll ever make."

"Touché," Elli smiled at her friend.

"Do you mind if I keep the drawing you made for me?" asked Cynthia.

"Sure!" Elli tore and folded the page from her planner, then handed it to Cynthia.

"Thanks friend!" Cynthia offered with the radiant sincerity of a friend as she took the notes.

"The pleasure was all mine! It really was! Call me after you meet with Rick tomorrow." Elli got into her car and started the engine.

"I will."

Two broad smiles departed the parking lot.

It ain't what you don't know that gets you into trouble.
It's what you know for sure that just ain't so.

— Mark Twain

Work Role Mastery

Outcomes   Resources

Risks

Attraction   Security   Agreement!

Are   Fulfillment   Do

meaning   pleasure

strengths

I

Ve   Effects

are   A Zone

FLOW

B Zone

do

Choice   Realization   Predictability

TWELVE

RENEWAL

C ynthia had been eager to get to work the next day. She could hardly sleep. During the night she had gotten up and made a list of the thoughts that were now flowing from her head. It was a longer and more comprehensive list than she expected. One thought begat another. It was strange, but she now had a new peacefulness. Even learning just a little about Relationship Performance had caused her to see everything about her work in a whole new light. She now understood why Rick might be ready to terminate her, and frankly, she felt fortunate that he hadn't done so already. "He must see something in me," she reflected to herself. More important-ly, she now had some real clues as to why her personal satis-faction at work had been so off track recently.

She was dumbfounded and, at the same time, appreci-ated that she had been clueless about so many of the big fac-tors and influences taking place every day at work. *Work's a we thing!* Her point of view combined more humility and confidence at the same time. How could that be? She now knew that the Organizational Triangle offered power to get what she needed and wanted from her work. She now had to rely upon this framework to get and keep her work at-tractive to an organization. She now appreciated the Orga-nizational Triangle as a powerful career magnet that attracts, or repels, supervisors and leaders to value and invest in any worker.

She also understood the Personal Triangle can be used to map and define personal work needs, aversions, and career wants. But first, she had to attend to securing her work role. Then she would use that security as a launch-ing pad for achieving the happiness and satisfaction she had been missing for so long at work, step by step. A lingering thought was in the back of her mind—was it too late? She really hoped it wasn't. On the way in she called Rick's assis-tant and was put on his calendar for 9 AM. "What a differ-ence a day can make," she thought as she found a smile on her face. Yeh, weird.

Once a problem is well understood, an elegant solution
is possible.
— Unknown

Rick was plowing through a screen full of e-mails as she walked in. "Hi Cynthia," he said in a friendly but pensive tone, still simultaneously perusing and trashing e-mails. He looked up briefly, "What's up?"

Cynthia was armed and ready. She pounced in and sat down in front of his desk like a tiger poised to leap. "Rick, I haven't been happy with my work lately. I also suspect you have not been at all satisfied with my work role performance either. Things have to change for both of us or this relationship just will not work out any longer."

"Wait a minute! Work role? Relationship? Performance?" Rick said, more than a little startled and actually shocked as he moved toward her, placing his elbows on the desk. He had been increasingly concerned about Cynthia's performance recently, and in fact had discussed taking action in a recent meeting. However, he had no idea that she too, was so frustrated. He felt the twinge and slight vertigo of being a bit out of control.

Cynthia had no doubt that she had captured his total attention now. "I met with my friend, Elli, last evening. She shared with me the basics of a practice they apply at her workplace called Relationship Performance, or RP for short. It's a philosophy that everybody accepts and uses to achieve the mission and to enjoy their work while doing it. RP is radically different from all the schemes and programs we've tried around here. It's far more powerful and practical than anything I have ever been exposed to before. It seems to largely be a way to apply better thinking, information and common sense in a practical, easy way. Relationship Performance puts a bright light on realities here that I did not understand before."

"What are we talking about? A training program, a book or something?"

"Nope, it's unique. If I understand correctly, there's a fast easy approach to getting RP underway by everyone using shared tools and discussion. There's a lot of flexibility in how you apply it. Central to its success is everyone accepting shared accountability for work performance from the top down."

"Alas, you've discovered yet another management fad, perhaps?" Rick offered with the combined sarcasm and skepticism that she too had offered earlier with Elli. She anticipated this, and was ready for doubts and prejudice.

"This is no fad, Rick. I was skeptical too, at least at first. Elli shared with me that this has become a cornerstone of her organization's competitive strategy. It's very serious and real. She described RP as 'unleashing the power of people, by design™' … as opposed to luck, trial and error or seat of the pants things like our dreaded performance reviews, useless worker satisfaction surveys, dubious training events and so forth."

"OK, I'm confused, but at least you've got me interested. You have 10 minutes." Rick looked at his watch, obviously interested, yet pulled to return to his morning e-mail.

Cynthia began, "RP explains how work really works, as well as what's happening when neither the needs of the organization or the worker are satisfied. As the name implies, it's all about constructing a solid performance-based relationship between the worker and the organization, so that each gain what they seek from work roles. The most radical thing is that it constantly reminds you that *work's a we thing* and that we each have shared accountability for getting what we want from the other. I'd never thought of it this way. It works by causing both workers and supervisors to accurately understand universal organizing principles that relate to all work roles. This allows each party to define their needs as well as what they have to offer to the other party. And you're going to like this Rick, everything centers on a measurable standard of work quality that's bi-directional," she emphasized *measurable* and *quality* to make sure Rick heard each of those words with crystal clarity.

She continued, "Whenever the level of quality isn't high enough for either party, there's a tool for structured, diagnostic dialog. After the dialog is over, there's a collaborative tool to form a sustainable agreement. This documents shared accountability to ensure that we both adhere to it. It's that simple—better thought, information, agreement

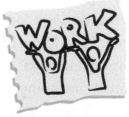

and accountability leads to better performance. It seems highly-effective and sustainable. RP is certainly very different than anything we're presently doing here."

"Well it's different all right. But dividing and sharing accountability for performance? I'm not sure I'd like that at all. I like to give orders with everyone saluting and then doing," he said with his kidding grin. Then he continued in a more serious tone, "but this is all a little overwhelming Cynthia, especially this early in the morning. I really wasn't expecting ..."

"I know, I would have never believed I'd be having this discussion with you 24 hours ago. But hear me out, Rick. Please ..."

"OK, but what's in this for our organization? You know the drill by now, Cynthia. Where's the ROI? It's all about ROI around here." Rick's skepticism was softening and now he was also honorably towing the company line.

"Precisely! That's the big point! RP has caused me to really see that, and in a more complete way. I have to provide you and our organization with better outcomes every day. Yes, much more than I have been offering the last few months. You have to get the maximum ROI from me, every day. I know this more clearly. And you have, and still are, investing a lot in me. I now better appreciate that fact too. I also know I have to do my work in a way that keeps the organization's resources that are invested in me to a minimum, including your own time and attention. You should never have to spend a moment worrying about me being at peak performance for our objectives. Additionally, I know that I must do everything I do at work in a way that minimizes risks. And lastly, I know that I have to do all of this better than any other option you may have to choose from, including your option of replacing me with another person down the street or overseas, or with some type of new software or robot. It's the only way I can have any security in my work role. It's the only way that work can work well and reliably for any worker. In sum, the rewards go straight to our bottom line." Even Cynthia was surprised by her energized remarks.

> *What lies behind us, and what lies before us are tiny*
> *matters compared to what lies within us.*
> — Ralph Waldo Emerson

Rick had begun making notes. That was a positive sign, she thought.

"Wow. Who are you?" Rick said, shaking his head and smiling. "After all these years, I'm not sure I know you, Cynthia! It's like someone else is in your body. How can I not like what you're proposing based on what I'm hearing. Outcomes? Resources? Risks? Be my best option? Frankly, I haven't even organized my thoughts like that before as to what I need, but you are speaking dead center to my bullseye of focus as a leader. It does appear that RP is language all of us supervisors need to be speaking around here."

"Well there's more. Lots more, for it's equally the language of workers. On the personal side of the work quality equation I, and all workers, have different and distinct needs, aversions and preferences too. I realize I'm bored and frustrated with what I am doing presently. But it's my responsibility to figure out where I am motivated and where I am not, what work role functions and circumstances I enjoy and what I need from my work. I have to know how to think this stuff through, then express it to you so we can meet each other's requirements to have better work in a better life. And you have a reason to listen because a worker always performs best doing what they enjoy and are truly motivated to do. Top performance and work enjoyment are two sides of the same coin! *My happiness at work can go straight to increasing our bottom line!*" Cynthia then braced herself for objections and pushback from Rick.

There was a long moment of silence.

Then he slowly and thoughtfully spoke. "I believe I can agree with that. It's a strange slant from anything I've ever heard, but I have to admit, I do agree, even speaking personally in my own role." Rick replied, positive and even more interested. "OK, so what is it you need?"

Cynthia thought to herself, this is better than she anticipated. "Well, keep in mind, I know just enough to be dangerous at this point because all of my education so far is from a friend. She's a leader who's accomplished amazing things in her organization with new techniques. But this is where I think I'm heading—I need tougher assignments in my role and then the reasonable autonomy with your support to get them done. I need to know better from you specifically what our toughest challenges are. I also need to know more of the *'whys' about what we are doing* so I can offer better thought and innovation in my contributions. I want to play a greater part in solving problems. I want to uncover hidden opportunities and problems that we don't know we have. I need to sink my teeth into mission critical projects and get them to the finish line on time. Lately, I've been bouncing around too much. I've been doing plenty of activities, many of them unnoticed, but accomplishing very little results."

"Bouncing around?" Rick interrupted. He was clearly caught off guard by the comment.

"Sure! Lately I've been doing too many busy-bee activities and checking them off the list. A list that changes its direction every day it seems. I never know why we are doing things the way we are and we never seem to be getting anything right for our customers. I don't like that. It's not good for me and it's not good for our organization. I want to be accountable. I want to know I serve a real purpose, that my work has meaning and that I offer real value around here. I can perform better if I'm focused, on track and on objective. That will be better for me, and I believe that it will be better for you. And lastly, I ask that you and I start using the RP tools."

"This is way too good to be true," Rick said as he leaned back in his chair, clearly trying his best to rapidly ponder the implications, ramifications … and downside

risks. Try as he might, he could not find the risks. But he could already envision a wide range of rewards.

"It does seem that way, doesn't it? But again, now that you put it this way, it all does seem to me like common sense. I guess that's the way it is with any big and important discovery. Obvious after the fact. Right?" Cynthia felt like she was an encouraging coach all of a sudden.

"Well, that's what they say."

"Let's make our relationship better, Rick, and let's both get more of what we want from the work role that you have me in. What do you say?" Cynthia shifted from being a coach to a sales pro going for the close.

"Well, you know that you are making me an offer that no sane supervisor could possibly refuse. How do we begin?"

"Elli said we begin practicing Relationship Performance by using something called *rpPaQ*™. I looked at the web site for it. You need to look at it too when your schedule permits. From what I understand, rpPaQ includes guidance, licensing and online tools that provide structure, process and information we each need for better thinking, dialog, agreement and monthly monitoring of our relationship. I'm fascinated with how it treats us both equally, prevents assumptions and offers each of us the same tools and support. If we choose to do this in a larger way with others here, we'll have something called *rpScoreboards*™ so everyone will know how our organization and each team is doing every month. We would share accountability and information to gain *better work in better lives.* Elli says there's no training required, but she strongly advised that having small, open, group discussions *before* using the tools is the best way to start practicing RP. There's a better explanation at the web site, so you might want to take a look at that too."

Cynthia went on, "Elli offered to have someone contact you today to make arrangements for getting things underway … assuming, of course, that you approve that we move forward on this. No training or consulting is required, but both are available should we prefer. Elli assures me that once we do this, we'll never look back at the old ways of doing things at work. In fact, at some point in time I might like to become certified in Relationship Performance and Talent Stewardship. That allows one to instruct and guide others in our organization as we put RP into even deeper practice by extending it into our work role design and strategic recruiting."

"OK, I get it. If I understand you correctly, this appears to be all upside and no down side. It sure sounds different. Maybe it's time for real improvements around here. Have Elli call me and I'll investigate this further." Rick still seemed a little off-balance and astounded at the personal transformation that was taking place. It was like some kind of a dream. But it was logical and real enough for him to know he had never experienced anything like this with any associate. Ever! This might be the real breakthrough that the organization really needed presently, he thought to himself. "What if every worker saw work like this? Thank you, Elli!"

"Roger, boss!" Cynthia offered a mock salute with a smile as she stood up, heading for the door.

"Cynthia?"

"Do you really think we could do this kind of thing with everyone here?"

"I believe we have to, Rick!" Cynthia said, feeling the big smile on her face, "After all, **Work's a We Thing!**"

A conclusion is where you got tired of thinking.
— Martin H. Fisher

Never promise more than you can perform.
— Publilus Syrus

AFTERWORD

The late Nicholas Hobbs offered counsel that I believe some readers will value as they strive to place thoughtfully chosen work roles into their lives.

—Danny

The Art of Getting into Trouble

Life is highly problematic, and what you become will rest in no small measure on the kinds of problem situations you get yourself into and have to work yourself out of. It is exceedingly difficult for a person to take thought and alter the quality and character and direction of his life. However, he can choose the direction he would like his life to take and then put himself deliberately in situations that will require the evolution of himself toward the kind of person he would like to become.

It is deep in the nature of man to make problems for himself. Man has often been called the problem-solver, but he is even more the problem-maker. Every noble achievement of men—in government, art, architecture, literature, and above all, in service—represents a new synthesis of the human experience, deepening our understanding and enriching our spirit. But each solid noble achievement creates new problems, often of unexpected dimension, and man moves eagerly on to face these new perplexities and to impose his order upon them. And so it will be, world without end. To know a person, it is useful to know what he has done, another way of defining what problems he has solved. It is even more informative, however, to know what problems he is working on now. For these will define the growing edge of his being.

We sometimes think of the well-adjusted person as having very few problems, while, in fact, just the opposite is true. When a person is ill or injured or crushed with grief or deeply frightened, the range of his concerns becomes sharply constructed; his problems diminish in scope and quality and complexity.

By contrast, the healthy in body and mind and spirit, is a person faced with many difficulties. He has a lot of problems, many of which he has deliberately chosen with the sure knowledge that in working toward their solution, he will become more the person he would like to be.

Part of the art of choosing difficulties is to select those that are indeed just manageable. If the difficulties chosen are too easy, life is boring; if they're too hard, life is self-defeating. The trick is to move oneself in the direction of what he would like to become at a level of difficulty close to the edge of his competence. When one achieves this fine tuning of his life, he will know zest and joy and deep fulfillment.

—Nicholas Hobbs from *The Art of Getting into Trouble*
Commencement Address, May 1968
Peabody Demonstration School, Nashville, TN

For book discussion guide
and additional resources visit:

www.rpPaQ.com